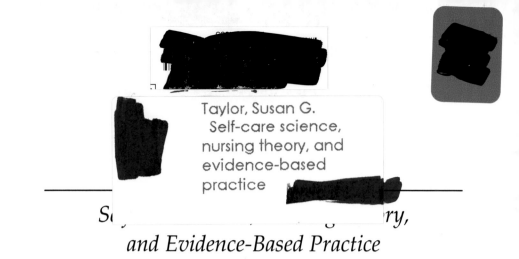

Taylor, Susan G.
 Self-care science,
nursing theory, and
evidence-based
practice

S...y, ...ry,
and Evidence-Based Practice

D0745780

Susan Gebhardt Taylor, MSN, PhD, FAAN, is Professor Emerita, Sinclair School of Nursing, University of Missouri–Columbia, Columbia, Missouri. Her bachelor's degree is from Alverno College, Milwaukee, Wisconsin, and her graduate degrees are from The Catholic University of America, Washington, DC. She is the recipient of the Alumna of the Year award from Alverno College, Missouri Tribute to Nurses–Nurse Educator award, Kemper Fellowship for Teaching Excellence, and MU Alumni Association Faculty award. She became an Honorary Alumnus of the Sinclair School of Nursing in 2009. Since retirement, she has kept active with the International Orem Society, American Association of Retired Persons, and Retired Seniors Volunteer Program, and serves on the board of directors of Primaris Healthcare Business Solutions.

Katherine Renpenning, MScN, is a nursing consultant particularly interested in the relationship between nursing theory and practice and education. She is a graduate of the University of Saskatchewan and the University of British Columbia. Early experiences in developing a curriculum in a school of nursing (1962), working with a research team in exploring the feasibility of a computerized patient record (1963), and developing a computerized application in nursing education (1974) led to a search for the answer to the questions "what is the focus of nursing, why do persons need nursing, how does one determine the content of a nursing course, and how does one determine the content of a patient record?" Direction for answering these questions was found in self-care deficit nursing theory and led to the consulting practice. Her client base has included governments, professional nursing associations, schools of nursing, and acute, long-term care, and community health agencies in Canada, the United States, and internationally.

Self-Care Science, Nursing Theory, and Evidence-Based Practice

Susan Gebhardt Taylor, MSN, PhD, FAAN

Katherine Renpenning, MScN

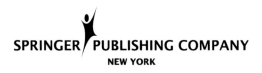

SPRINGER PUBLISHING COMPANY
NEW YORK

Springer Publishing Company, LLC
11 West 42nd Street
New York, NY 10036
www.springerpub.com

Acquisitions Editor: Margaret Zuccarini
Senior Editor: Rose Mary Piscitelli
Composition: S4Carlisle Publishing Services

ISBN 978-0-8261-0778-7
E-book ISBN: 978-0-8261-0779-4

11 12 13 14/ 5 4 3 2 1

The author and the publisher of this Work have made every effort to use sources believed to be reliable to provide information that is accurate and compatible with the standards generally accepted at the time of publication. Because medical science is continually advancing, our knowledge base continues to expand. Therefore, as new information becomes available, changes in procedures become necessary. We recommend that the reader always consult current research and specific institutional policies before performing any clinical procedure. The author and publisher shall not be liable for any special, consequential, or exemplary damages resulting, in whole or in part, from the readers' use of, or reliance on, the information contained in this book. The publisher has no responsibility for the persistence or accuracy of URLs for external or third-party Internet Web sites referred to in this publication and does not guarantee that any content on such Web sites is, or will remain, accurate or appropriate.

Library of Congress Cataloging-in-Publication Data
Taylor, Susan G.
  Self-care science, nursing theory, and evidence-based practice / Susan
Gebhardt Taylor, Katherine Renpenning.
      p.; cm.
  ISBN 978-0-8261-0778-7 — ISBN 978-0-8261-0779-4 (e-book)
  1. Self-care, Health. 2. Evidence-based nursing. 3. Nursing.
  I. Renpenning, Kathie. II. Title.
  [DNLM: 1. Self Care. 2. Evidence-Based Nursing.
  3. Nursing Care—methods. 4. Nursing Theory. WB 327]
  RA776.95.T39 2011
  610.73—dc22

                                                    2011004867

Printed in the United States of America by Gasch Printing

Contents

Preface

To our knowledge, this book is the first of its kind. It clearly establishes the link between evidence-based nursing practice, nursing theory, and the foundational nursing sciences, including the science of self-care. There are two international trends in health care that led to our deciding to write this book—self-care and evidence-based practices. We have been committed to self-care as it relates to nursing for decades. Interest in the concept of self-care is taking on broader appeal, so much so that there is not at present a clear understanding of what it is.

The sciences of self-care and nursing as presented in this text have their origin in work done by the nursing theorist Dorothea Orem. For more than 40 years Orem has recognized, spoken, and written of the need for nursing to develop the science base of nursing practice. In 1993, Orem invited a small international group of nurses, which became known as the Orem Study Group, to meet with her to further the development of self-care deficit nursing theory. We began the work with discussion about the discipline of nursing and nursing science. Two major products of the group activity, which have guided development of this text, are the structure of the discipline (Figure 1.4) and a schematic representation of the nursing practice sciences (Figure 1.5).

There is a science of self-care that goes beyond people doing things for themselves. The current movement toward evidence-based nursing is leading to serious discourse regarding the meaning of knowledge and evidence in nursing. To have an evidence-based view of practice, the professional nurse needs to have a clear frame of reference regarding the proper object of nursing and the structure of the discipline in order to frame the problem. The science of self-care and the related sciences, including the nursing-specific knowledge as expressed in the self-care deficit nursing theory developed and promulgated by Dorothea Orem and others, provides the structure and content for understanding self-care. In this book, we consider the science of self-care, the constituent foundational nursing sciences, and the practical nursing sciences as the basis for evidence-based practice and education.

Susan Gebhardt Taylor, MSN, PhD, FAAN
Katherine Renpenning, MScN

Acknowledgments

First, we would like to recognize 25 stimulating and exciting years of working with Dorothea Orem without whose guidance, inspiration, and contributions this book would never have come about. We want to acknowledge the contributions of the following to the continuing development of self-care deficit nursing theory: the Nursing Development Conference Group, the Orem Study Group, and the International Orem Society. We would be remiss in not recognizing the ongoing work of faculties of schools of nursing, and the individual scholars and practitioners around the world who continue to make significant contributions to theory development and related nursing practice.

We are grateful to Barbara Banfield for reading drafts as the book took shape. Her knowledge of the theory makes her a leading expert. We appreciate Elizabeth Geden for sharing her practical wisdom.

Thank you to all who have made this book a reality.

Susan and Kathie

I

Self-Care Science and Nursing Theory

*T*his book is concerned with two themes that are prominent in to-day's nursing literature: evidence-based practice and self-care. The purpose of the book is to explore new ways of looking at the inter-relationship of these topics from the perspective of nursing practice. Theory and science are necessary and linked parts of the development of the discipline of nursing.

Section I begins with a discussion of the proper object or focus of the discipline of nursing (the reason for the existence of the nursing profession). This focus is identified as persons who are unable to provide for themselves the amount and quality of self-care required to maintain life, health, and promote development. Accepting this leads to exploring the question: if this is the proper object of the discipline, what are the questions of concern to nursing and what constitutes evidence for nursing purposes? Through identification of variables associated with the performance of self-care operations and hypothesizing about the relationships of those variables, a foundation for a science of self-care has evolved.

The science of self-care and the nursing practice sciences are linked in the production of nursing action by providing a theoretical framework derived from a science of self-care for clinical decision making by the nurse. Furthermore, the nursing theory uses a science of self-care that is interdisciplinary and is used internationally. Persons interested in health-related self-care regardless of their specific discipline need to know how to determine efficacy of actions taken or proposed, and how to assist clients in developing capabilities in relation to self-care. Development of these professions and disciplines rely on a science of self-care which goes beyond the common sense view or the medically related view of self-care.

The science of self-care identifies what a person requires to be healthy, the complexity of factors that change or modify these requirements, the actions a person takes to maintain their health and well-being, and limitations in the individual's ability to take action. It also includes the self-care systems used or needed by persons experiencing a change in health-state or environment. Though the initial focus is on explicating a science of self-care that is individually based, the science also presents components that explain the relationship of self-care to dependents, family, community, and culture.

Chapter 1 focuses on the development of the self-care deficit theory of nursing as the basis for the discipline of nursing and the conceptual elements of the nursing theory, including the science of self-care. This is further explored in Chapter 2. The following chapters continue to develop and expand the concepts presented in the theory of nursing and the science of self-care. Section II then describes the practice science of nursing derived from, or associated with, the science and theory of self-care and nursing.

1

The Proper Object of Nursing and a Theory of Nursing Practice

Self-care is work. It is work required by or for every person to maintain life and health as well as to promote development. When persons are unable to provide the quantity and quality of self-care required, they need assistance. If this assistance is beyond the common sense knowledge acquired by the family or other lay caregivers in any society, the assistance of specially prepared caregivers is required. These categories of specialized caregivers are known by the specialized services they provide. From the self-care deficit nursing theory perspective, the care or assistance provided by the nurse is associated with health-related actual or potential self-care deficits of persons, individually or collectively.

An explicit relationship between nursing and self-care was first made by Orem in 1956. Since then, under her leadership and guidance, that connection has been developed into a general theory of nursing, the *self-care deficit nursing theory*. The theory explains why people require nursing care, the processes for the production of the required care, and a structure for the development of the sciences of self-care, the practical sciences of nursing, and the related knowledge associated with these sciences.

A NURSING PRACTICE THEORY WITH FOUR PARTS

The self-care deficit nursing theory is a nursing practice theory with four parts. The first and major component is the *theory of nursing systems.* The theory of nursing systems encompasses both the *theory of self-care* and the *theory of self-care deficits.* The *theory of self-care* refers to the requirements for self-care and the powers and capabilities of the person to provide this care. The *theory of self-care deficits* reflects an imbalance between the required self-care and ability to perform the care. The identification of the existence or potential for a self-care deficit associated with health is the basis for establishing the nursing system. The fourth and last part is the corollary *theory of dependent care* which presents elements related to caring for persons who are socially dependent. Figure 1.1 shows the relationship among the four parts of this nursing practice theory.

The variables of concern for nursing practice are the components of the theories, defined in Exhibit 1.1 and elaborated further in the book.

What is the condition that exists in a person when judgments are made that a nurse(s) should be brought into the situation? It is obvious that not everyone is in need of the services of a nurse all the time. Nurses possess knowledge and skills that any person can benefit from at some time, but are not required, or even desirable, all the time. So what is the basis for judgments about a need for nursing? It is "the inability of persons to provide continuously for themselves the amount and quality of required self-care because of situations of personal health" (Orem, 2001, p. 20). This statement is elegant, each word is significant

FIGURE 1.1   Relationship of the Four Parts of Self-Care Deficit Nursing Theory

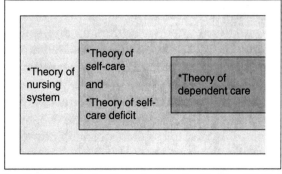

Source: Adapted from D. E. Orem, *Nursing: Concepts of Practice,* 6th ed., p. 141 (St. Louis, MO: Mosby, 2001). Copyright Orem estate, used with permission of Walene E. Shields, heir of Dorothea E. Orem.

EXHIBIT 1.1
Variables of Concern for Practice and the Definitions

Therapeutic self-care demand summarizes all of the action required over time to meet known self-care requisites. A self-care requisite expresses the goals of action necessary for regulating an aspect(s) of human functioning and development. There are three categories of self-care requisites or goals of self-care: *universal*, which are common to all persons; *developmental*, which are particular to the person's developmental stage; and *health deviation*, which address particular health states.

Self-care agency is persons' ability to know and meet their continuing requirements for self-care in order to regulate their own human functioning and development. It is a threefold construct that includes:

1. Self-care operations of knowing, decision making, and acting with the abilities associated with each operation.
2. The operations are derived from action theory.
3. The 10 power components, which are abilities specific to self-care.

Capabilities and dispositions are foundational to deliberate action.

Dependent-care agency is the "capabilities of persons to know and meet the therapeutic self-care demands of persons socially dependent on them or to regulate the development or exercise of these persons' self-care ability" (Orem, 1995, p. 457).

Dependent-care deficit is a relational statement and describes the relationship between the self-care deficit of the dependent (the required assistance) and dependent-care agency (the capabilities of the care provider). Identification of a dependent-care deficit indicates a need for further assistance.

Nursing agency is "the developed capabilities of persons educated as nurses that empowered them to represent themselves as nurses and within the frame of a legitimate interpersonal relationship to act, to know, and to help persons in such relationships to meet their therapeutic self-care demands and regulate the development or exercise of their self-care agency" (Orem, 2001, p. 518).

Nursing systems are series and sequences of deliberate practical actions of nurses performed at times in coordination with actions of their patients . . . (Orem, 2001, p. 519).

———————
Definitions used with permission of Orem's estate administrator.

and it expresses the whole of nursing. It leads to many insights and questions, all of which give direction to the foundation of practice, research, and knowledge development. For example, "inability" moves us to ask what are the expected abilities a person needs to be able to care for self; what is the level, degree, or nature of these limitations? How might one develop these abilities? What factors could

FIGURE 1.2   A Conceptual Framework for Nursing

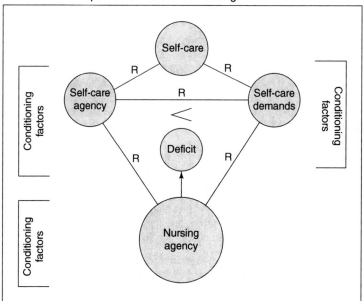

Source: Reprinted from D. E. Orem, *Nursing: Concepts of Practice,* 6th ed., p. 491 (St. Louis, MO: Mosby, 2001). Used with permission of Walene E. Shields, heir of Dorothea E. Orem.

influence or affect the person's ability to care for self or for others, for example, infants, children, elderly, and the chronically ill? As Orem and others worked to answer these kinds of questions, the basic structure of the self-care deficit nursing theory was made known as a nursing practice theory with four parts. The basic conceptual elements are shown in Figure 1.2, a conceptual framework for nursing (Orem, 2001, p. 491). The self-care deficit nursing theory is comprised of the patient variables of self-care/dependent-care agency and therapeutic self-care demand/dependent-care demand; the nurse variable, that is, nursing agency, and the relationships between them. All of these are described in detail in the later chapters.

NURSING: A PROFESSION AND A DISCIPLINE

Nursing is both a profession and a discipline. Nursing as a field of practice is a profession; as a field of knowledge, nursing is a discipline. Although distinct entities, in a practice discipline they are in reality inseparable— as the saying goes "you can't have one without the other."

FIGURE 1.3   Relationship of Profession to Discipline

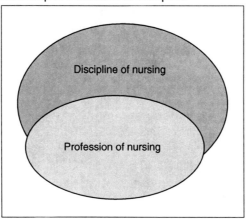

The profession of nursing relies on the discipline of nursing to inform the practice, to provide the knowledge that is transformed into practice, useful in designing systems of nursing for individual persons or groups, and for developing institutional systems for delivery of care. And while the discipline of nursing provides the knowledge base for practice, ever expanding or clarifying the understanding of the theoretical or science base for practice, practice experiences give direction to the development of theoretical knowledge. There is knowledge needed for the profession that is outside the disciplinary knowledge, such as knowledge of specific political systems affecting the work environment (Figure 1.3).

A *profession* is an *occupationally related social institution* established and maintained as a means of providing essential services to the individual and the society. Some commonly accepted characteristics of a profession include the following. Each profession is concerned with an identified area of need or function, for example, maintenance of physical and emotional health, preservation of rights and freedom, enhancing the opportunity to learn. Professionals are assumed to have extensive theoretical knowledge and to possess skills based on that knowledge that they are able to apply in practice. The profession collectively, and the professional individually, possesses a body of knowledge and a repertoire of behaviors and skills (professional culture) needed in the practice of the profession; such knowledge, behavior, and skills normally are not possessed by the nonprofessional. In some professions, the body of knowledge is relatively inaccessible to the uninitiated. Nursing has as one of its goals making the knowledge and skills of the profession more accessible.

Professional knowledge contains elements that cannot be communicated in the form of rules and can only be acquired through experience. Members of the profession are involved in decision making in the service of the client. These decisions are made in accordance with the most valid knowledge available, against a background of principles and theories, and within the context of possible impact on other related conditions or decisions. The current movement toward evidence-based practice is an effort to meet this professional characteristic. A profession is based on one or more undergirding disciplines from which it builds its own basic and applied knowledge and skills (Wikipedia, http://www.adprima.com/profession.htm).

The body of nursing knowledge referred to in the characteristics of profession is the discipline of nursing. A *discipline* is a *structured body of knowledge* about a particular segment of reality. "Each discipline has a unique focus for knowledge development that directs its inquiry and distinguishes it from other fields" (Smith & Liehr, 2008, p. 1). The structure of that knowledge serves as a matrix for examining relationships between theoretical and practical concepts and propositions. It presents to the scholar/researcher/practitioner a view of gaps in knowledge within the field and areas where new knowledge, developed through various accepted methods, articulates with current knowledge.

The discipline of nursing is seen by some scholars (Fawcett, 2000) as having an over-arching structure or metaparadigm comprised of four major elements: *person, environment, health, and nursing.* The particular definition of each element gives room for variation in general theories or models of nursing. These elements were derived in the 1970–1980s from existing theories of nursing and did not influence the initial direction of development of self-care deficit nursing theory though they are evident in the theory. The definitions presented here are congruent with self-care deficit nursing theory conceptualizations.

Person, or human being, refers to both the recipient of care and the giver of care. Detailed in Chapters 1 and 2, human beings are unitary beings who exist in their environments. Self-care deficit nursing theory includes the whole reality of human beings, singly and in social units as the material object of nursing. This includes individuals, dependent units, and multi-person units such as families and communities and their relationship to nursing as a profession and as a discipline.

It includes persons who occupy the position or fill the role of nurse. "A nurse is one who knows nursing and can and does produce it" (Orem, 2001, p. 40).

The person and *environment* within which persons exist are inseparable but factors about the environment and human relationship can be isolated and described. From the view of self-care deficit nursing theory, a significant meaning of environment is as a basic conditioning factor, the meaning of which is described in Chapter 2. Environment conditions the persons' need for self-care, the actions selected and the setting within which care is given, the opportunity to engage in those actions, and the restricting influences which interfere with that engagement. There are physical, chemical, biologic, social, and political features. Culture is an element of environment. Further references are made to the meaning of environment throughout the text.

Health refers to the state of wholeness of structure and function of a living person. There are two dominant themes in the many definitions of health that have meaning for self-care deficit nursing theory. The first is that evidence of holistic integrated functioning and evaluative judgments about health or not-health can be made by the self or others. Much of this evidence can be objectively measured; others can be identified by observation or self-report. Second, individuals have their own sense of health and well-being, their own definitions of health formed within a cultural context. Orem distinguishes between health and well-being. Well-being relates to the second theme, that of the individual's subjective views, whereas health is the more objective determination based on evidence of integrated structure and functioning. What persons understand as health and what they value as to the functioning and integrity of the self affects the persons' self-care as much as does the evidence of integrated functioning. This is further explored in Chapter 4.

Nursing is an essential human service; the definitive characterizing structure of nursing is made known through a general theory of nursing. Nursing is produced in a particular time and a particular place through discrete deliberate actions or sequences of actions. Nursing exists through relationship of nurse and patient and what they choose to do. The self-care deficit nursing theory is a theory about the variables of concern when the service of nursing is required as nurses and patient interact, and about the variations in relationships among those variables. The basic conceptual elements are shown in Figure 1.2, a conceptual framework for nursing as described previously. At its most elemental, self-care deficit nursing theory is comprised of two patient variables—self-care agency and therapeutic self-care demand, one nurse variable, nursing agency, and the relationship between the nurse and patient.

THE STRUCTURE OF NURSING SCIENCE

Originally, science was synonymous with knowledge (from the Latin *scientia*, meaning knowledge). As knowledge expanded and ways of thinking and generalizing about us and the world around us became more elaborate and expansive, science took on a more specific meaning. Science, in its broadest sense, is "any systematic knowledge that is capable of resulting in a correct prediction or reliable outcome. This comes about through observation, study, and experimentation carried on to determine the nature or principles of what is being studied. In its more restricted sense, science is a system of acquiring knowledge based on scientific method, and the organized body of knowledge gained through such research. In this sense science is a systematic enterprise of gathering knowledge about the world and organizing and condensing that knowledge into testable laws and theories" (Wikipedia, http://en.wikipedia.org/wiki/Science). Referred to as natural or empirical sciences, this knowledge must be based on observable phenomena and capable of being tested for its validity by other researchers working under the same conditions.

In recent years the category "human science" has emerged, referring to "a philosophy and approach to science that seeks to understand human experience in deeply subjective, personal, historical, contextual, cross-cultural, political, and spiritual terms. Human science is the science of qualities rather than of quantities and closes the subject-object split in science. It is interpretive, reflective, and appreciative" (Wikipedia, http://en.Wikipedia.org/wiki/human_science). Others classify sciences as basic and applied. Basic sciences are empirical, theoretical sciences, whereas applied sciences take the findings of the basic sciences and, literally, apply them in a practical manner to solve a problem. All of these descriptions or categories of science have validity and utility for nursing knowledge development.

Nursing is a practical science. In 1969, Simon proposed the science of the artificial. He stated that "certain phenomena are 'artificial' in a very specific sense: They are as they are only because of a system's being molded, by goals or purposes, to the environment in which it lives . . . artificial phenomena have an air of 'contingency' in their malleability by environment" (p. ix). Viewing nursing as an "artificial" science helped Orem and the Nursing Development Conference Group (NDCG) develop the self-care deficit theory of nursing. Artificial, meaning produced by art rather than nature, refers to things made by persons, not necessarily material, characterized in terms of functions, goals, and adaptations. Simon found the artificial to be "interesting principally when it concerns complex systems that live in complex environments" (Simon, 1969, p. xi). Simon provided NDCG with that and many other insights that aided them in their development of the theory of nursing systems and the science of design which he called "the core of all professional training." At that same time, Argyris and colleagues were developing theories of practice and actions science (Argyris, Putnam, & Smith, 1985; Argyris & Schön, 1974). They presented ideas related to problem framing or setting, that is, when one "select[s] the problem, we select what we will treat as the 'things' of the situation, we set the boundaries of our attention to it, and we impose upon it a coherence which allows us to say what is wrong and in what directions the situation needs to be changed" (Schön, 1983, p. 40). Other important concepts introduced were that of the interrelationship of scientist and practitioner and reflection and learning. Though these ideas were overshadowed by the increasing favor of the empirical sciences related to the natural, leading to a focus on the relevant nonnursing sciences as identified in Figure 1.4, the structures of the disciplines such as physiology and sociology are emerging amid the discourse regarding evidence and evidence-based nursing.

Early in the process of developing self-care deficit nursing theory, the NDCG identified nursing as a *practical science*, that is, one of action, behavior and conduct with speculative and practical knowledge (NDCG, 1979, 2nd ed., p. 105). A practical science seeks to produce or construct its object and needs scientific knowledge to do so. Practical science has theoretic and speculative parts, as well as parts that give direction to what to do or what not to do in distinct situations. Practical sciences include speculatively practical knowledge and practically practical knowledge, whereas the theories and conceptual elements of self-care deficit nursing theory are speculative in mode (Orem, 2001, p. 164).

Within the discipline of nursing there are categories of nursing science. These are named and the relationships shown in Figure 1.4. This figure indicates points at which knowledge from other disciplines can inform nursing knowledge and vice versa.

12

FIGURE 1.4 The Structure of the Discipline of Nursing

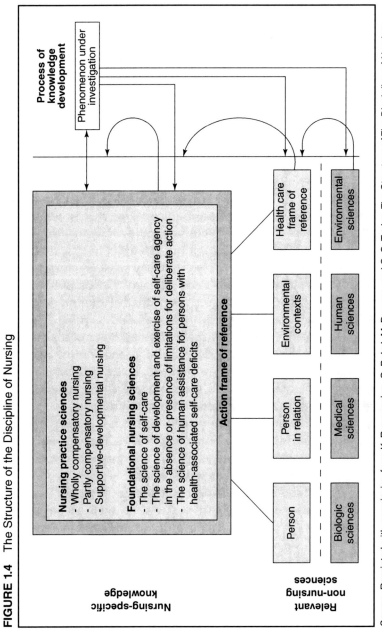

Source: Reprinted with permission from K. Renpenning, G. Bekel, M. Denyes, and S. G. Taylor, *The Structure of The Discipline of Nursing* (Germany, Ulm, 2004).

THE PROPER OBJECT OF NURSING

The critical issue regarding the development of the body of knowledge of nursing is identification and explication of the object of nursing, material and proper. As noted above, a discipline is a structured body of knowledge about a particular segment of reality. Paley (2010) described a network of theories, evidence, and models connected to adjacent nodes of the network, with each consequently reinforcing the whole structure. He described the ideas in a single location as having ramifications in all directions, and proposed that substantive changes a location can have repercussions even in distantly connected regions of the network.

This view of discipline moves from that of a hierarchical or pyramidal structure to one of a web with nodes and interconnections. Although models presenting the structures and substructures of the self-care deficit nursing theory are shown as two dimensional, they are best thought of as at least three-dimensional models.

The focus of a discipline is constituted by its object, which is a theoretical concept. The object of nursing is the human person. The proper or specific object of a discipline defines it; it designates the particular aspect of reality that is the subject of the discipline as it can be known and expressed. Though initially the boundaries and matrices of the discipline may be lacking in detail and the relationships of substance to matrix not yet established; over time the details become clearer and the design takes shape. Like creating a patchwork quilt, you begin with little pieces, sewing them together into blocks, eventually joining those separate blocks with sashing. As the sewer goes on, the design of the quilt becomes visible to others. Different sewers can add to the quilt or change and improve the design.

KNOWLEDGE DEVELOPMENT WITHIN A DISCIPLINE

The methods of developing the substantive knowledge of nursing include philosophical and scientific as well as other ways of knowing as described by scholars (Carper, 1978; Chinn & Kramer, 1999). Though many disciplines share the common object of the human person, they vary as to the aspect of person that forms the proper object and the different ways of knowing and types of knowledge accepted by the discipline. Differences and similarities in disciplines are necessary because each discipline does not cover all of reality; it is not global (Bekel, 1998, pp. 1–4). Recognizing boundaries and limitations for a discipline does not mean closed systems but does provide for identification of overlaps, areas where integrated knowledge may develop. It facilitates discourse between disciplines as well as within each discipline. The description of the object builds the center of professional endeavor of a discipline. The use of *proper object* to designate the focus of nursing was first used by Orem in 1958 (Orem, 2001, p. 20). The whole reality of human beings cared for, either singly or in social units, constitutes the material object of the activities of all the human services. Identification of the proper object, what distinguishes one field from another, includes "specification of various aspects of object domains as a way of describing how sciences use the identified object in the development of scientific disciplines, notably (a) problem domain, (b) application domain, (c) proper object domain, and (d) universe of discourse" (Weingartner, 1999, pp. 2–3). The proper object domain of *nursing* is found in the answer to the question as to what condition exists in a person when judgments are made that a nurse(s) should be brought into the situation, that is, those persons should be under nursing care. Orem asked the questions "Why do people need nursing, or what human condition brings about a need for nursing? What is nursing? What is the *structure* of the entity, that service we refer to as nursing?" (Orem, 1996, p. 302). For Orem, the answer was "the inability of persons to provide continuously for themselves the amount and quality of required self-care because of situations of personal health" (Orem, 2001, p. 20). Further responses to this question in the form of clarification, insights, formulations, and expressions provide the conceptual foundation for the body of work known as the self-care deficit nursing theory. Through the years there has been further development, clarification, elaboration, and verification in all levels of abstraction, including specific situation theory for practice.

HISTORY OF NURSING THEORY

What Is Past Is Prologue

The work done by nurses through the centuries is all essential work and is linked to contemporary nursing knowledge. Theorizing is a matter of proposing solutions, parameters, limitations. The natural inquisitiveness of humans leads them to ask questions and to seek solutions to situations encountered, to try to explain the reality they perceive within the limits of what is known, and to speculate about possibilities.

There has been theorizing about self-care and nursing since social groups first assigned specific persons the responsibility of taking care of members of the group who might be in need of assistance with daily care. The leaders of the group had to consider questions as to what personal actions are to be taken, for example, what to eat, how to do bodily care, where and when to sleep, what are acceptable activities? What is to be done for the injured hunter or warrior, ill children, elderly members? Who are the persons to whom the responsibility of assisting others is given? What are they expected to do? What are they allowed to do to another to meet the expectations? What are the consequences if they don't meet these expectations? The answers to these questions are found in the traditions and rules of the various groups. This kind of thinking laid the foundation for the evolution and development of organized care, both medicine and nursing. Select persons are assigned social tasks for caring for others, maintaining health. They begin to work out ways of doing things, reasons for taking a certain action over another. Special locations for caring for the ill were established, for example, *Hopital Hotel Dieu*, 660 A.D. in Paris. Like many early hospitals, it started as a general institution catering to the poor and sick, offering food and shelter in addition to medical care. In 1633 in France, Louise de Marillac began a systematic training of women, particularly for the care of the sick. In 1833 in Germany, Pastor Theodore Fleidner founded an order of deaconesses at Kaiserswerth to train nurses for hospital work. The content of the training programs identified the knowledge and skills believed at that time to be necessary for providing care to those sick and needy. Further comments on the history of nursing theory development are in Appendix A.

The efforts of these and other nurses led, inevitably, to the development of theoretical systems of nursing knowledge and practice. For what is theorizing but contemplation and offering explanations that eventually lead to a coherent group of propositions, a particular conception or view of something to be done and the method of doing it? And what is the purpose of theorizing in practice disciplines but the development of knowledge and science leading to practice based in empirical and personal evidence.

HISTORY OF SELF-CARE DEFICIT NURSING THEORY

Self-care deficit nursing theory is an important component of nursing's theoretical knowledge. This theory was first articulated in the 1950s, formalized and first published in 1972 for the purpose of laying out the structure of nursing knowledge and explicating the domains of nursing knowledge. Self-care deficit nursing theory was one of the first models of nursing developed. (Detailed presentations of the history of self-care deficit nursing theory can be found in Orem, 2001, Appendix B, 6th edition; Renpenning & Taylor, 2003, pp. 254–266; Taylor, 1997, pp. 7–10). Scholars wishing to learn more about the early work can access the Orem Archives at The Alan Mason Chesney Medical Archives of the Johns Hopkins Medical Institutions.

Orem identified two phases in the development of the theory. The first ended in 1972 when the essential ideas were identified, relationships described, and the first book was published: *Nursing: Concepts of Practice*. The second phase began in 1972, when the focus was on diffusion and refinement, and ended with her death in 2007. A new phase, or a continuation of the second phase, now focuses on research to validate theoretical relationships and the use of the theory in practice.

Dorothea Orem: The Person

Knowing some personal history lays the foundation for understanding her work. Orem, born in 1914, was one of two sisters who grew up in Baltimore, Maryland. In a personal interview in 1997, Orem described herself as early in her life having "a natural talent for seeing order and relationships especially with ideas and concepts and meanings" (Taylor, 1997). Reading was important to her from early on. Dorothea attended Seton High School in Baltimore. She recalls as most helpful the courses in English "We did a lot of analysis. We took things apart; we searched for meaning."

Her early exposure to nursing through her family made it a viable career choice for her. Nursing was chosen because of "practical reasons." When Orem decided to apply for nursing school, she chose Providence School of Nursing at Providence Hospital, Washington, DC, where her aunt was then supervisor of the operating room.

Orem did her preservice education at Providence Hospital during the depression. She received her diploma in nursing in 1934. She described some of her experiences in nursing school as helping to conceptualize order and relationships. She described two experiences that were a motivating force in developing and being able to express a concept of nursing, in both instances she saw what to her was "good nursing."

After receiving her diploma, Orem worked in the operating room, for 1 year. Experiences in the operating room helped her see the "whole picture" especially in terms of organization and administration. She did private duty nursing, in home and hospital, (there were no ICUs in those days) and staff nursing in pediatrics and adult medical/surgical units. She was evening supervisor in the emergency room, where she saw the articulations between nursing and practically everything else.

> Physicians and nurses worked together but the nurse was not under the physician in any sense of the word. There was collaborating with orders, but even with orders you had to know what you could and couldn't do. I think sometimes the burden on nurses is extreme because they have to know what's within limits of both fields—nursing and medicine. (Taylor, personal interview, 1997)

During this time she was going to The Catholic University of America (CUA) where she received her baccalaureate degree in 1939. She moved to Detroit in 1940 where she taught biological sciences at Providence Hospital School of Nursing. She returned to DC and took a position at Providence School of Nursing as assistant to the director of the program—then a combination of the old Providence program and CUA—where she taught a microbiology class. Orem received a master's degree in 1946. At that time the degree required a foreign language, German, and a thesis. Orem did her thesis work in the area of guidance. "It took me a long time to do that thesis, to find something to do." She returned to Detroit in 1945 as director of nursing service and director of the school of nursing. While there, she took a course in metaphysics at University of Detroit, a Jesuit university, a course that was important as a broad general tool in dealing with the matter of sorting and structuring the content of nursing, in reaching understanding, and in understanding both the parts and the whole as such. At that point she recognized that without a conceptualization of nursing, there are certain questions that can't be answered and one is therefore oriented to doing.

In 1949, Orem went to the Indiana State Board of Health, Hospital Division, to help in upgrading of nursing services in general hospitals.

There she noted that nurses had difficulty representing their needs to hospital administrators because they didn't know how to talk about nursing. She became focused on expressing what nursing is.

The mid-1950s was a time when there was beginning to be a focus on planning nursing care. Orem became aware that the "point of departure for planning care had to be the patient" not the nurses' tasks. "Then, another experience was when in the profession they put all this emphasis on planning your nursing care. The question that I asked is 'what is the basis for planning? What are you planning?' To me, there wasn't anything."

Following this time in Indiana, Orem returned to DC and took a position with the Office of Education, Vocational Section of the Technical division, where there was an on-going project to upgrade practical nurse training. It was at this time that the more formal work of structuring nursing knowledge began. "In my thinking that started at that time, I came to the conclusion that the question that had to be answered was 'why do people need nursing?' and her answer was that it is the inability of the person to maintain self-care in health situation." "From that time onward, the knowledge I had about nursing began to structure itself; the pieces started to come together" albeit with considerable work, alone and with others. Some of the elements of what is now known as self-care deficit nursing theory emerged and are recorded in *Guides for Developing Curricula for the Education of Practical Nurses* where she expressed the object of nursing.

After the publication of the guidelines, Orem returned to a faculty position at CUA in 1959. While there she began working on a book, *Foundations of Nursing* which was later self-published. Orem provided the intellectual leadership in developing self-care deficit nursing theory throughout the collaborative endeavors with members of the Nursing Models Committee at Catholic University of America, and the "Improvement in Nursing (IN) group," later the Nursing Development Conference Group (NDCG) comprised of nurses from all fields, including educators, administrators, and clinicians. After the publication of the first edition of *Nursing: Concepts of Practice* in 1971, Orem continued to work on the development of the theory. She consulted extensively and did many presentations at conferences. These often brought together the major theorists; however, there was little substantive interaction among them. Later Orem gathered a group of scholars, the Orem Study Group, to work with her in the development of the theory. Much of the work of this group is included in this book.

ROLE OF THEORY IN THE DEVELOPMENT
OF NURSING KNOWLEDGE

The relationship of nursing theory, research and practice is described in detail by many. Of note is the work of Young, Taylor, and Renpenning (2001). They identified two major outcomes of nursing theoretical systems. First, there is scientific, systematized knowledge for nursing practice that can also be used in designing research and curriculum. The second is a formalized statement of a philosophical worldview on which to base further understanding of nursing theory. Theory instructs the nurse in focus and content of that practice as well as guides nursing action. Theory informs practice and practice informs theory (Alligood & Tomey, 2002, p. 3). The same can be said about theory and research. In fact, the theoretical system provides a unifying focus for approaching a wide range of nursing concerns (Neuman & Fawcett, 2011). A conceptual model, such as self-care deficit nursing theory, can unify a number of middle-range theories and give direction to areas for further development. "Results from atheoretical studies or those that have no nursing theoretical link cannot be easily incorporated into the structure of nursing knowledge, and are at risk for losing their identity as nursing studies" (Kolcaba & Kolcaba, 2011, p. 307). Sieloff and Frey (2007) commented that

> Developing and testing propositions and formulations from nursing theory are critical for the development of nursing science. This process is also one of the most difficult approaches to knowledge building to establish and maintain. A primary reason for this may be the lack of support for nursing theories within the discipline . . . doctoral programs rarely require the use of an explicit nursing theory for dissertation work. (2007, p. xv)

Orem believed that general theories are not static but rather guide the work of scholars, practitoners, and researchers leading to refinement and further understandings. The more developed the conceptual model, the more meaningful the translation to specific situations recognizing that this knowledge is most useful when generalizations can be made within the context of the broader theory. Using self-care deficit nursing theory generates a style of thinking and a way of communicating nursing. A deeper way of thinking and interacting occurs when there is a shared language. It is both more effective and efficient; fewer misunderstandings and errors occur and less time is spent in clarifying meaning.

THE STRUCTURE OF THE DISCIPLINE OF NURSING

In designing the structure of the discipline of nursing, the Orem Study Group worked from the premise that all knowledge is ultimately related; though each discipline has a particular proper object, knowledge has meaning across boundaries. Knowledge development for the discipline and the practice of nursing is, or should be, built upon existing knowledge and integrated into existing bodies of knowledge. A broader view of nursing places it in the context of the world of human endeavor. Given the proper object of nursing as described, the Study Group examined the nature of persons and persons in relations. Nursing specific knowledge is framed within an action frame of reference as shown in Figure 1.4. The relevant non-nursing sciences provide the content for that frame of reference. It is the foundational nursing sciences and the nursing practice sciences that constitute nursing's unique body of knowledge. Though not specifically identified, Orem anticipated the development of a number of nursing applied sciences.

The philosophical view of human beings underlying the self-care deficit nursing theory is that human beings are unitary beings who exist in their environments. They are in a developmental process, striving to achieve their human potential and self-ideal through these processes. They possess free will and are capable of maintaining an awareness of self and environment. Human beings attach meaning to what is experienced, reflect upon their experiences, and possess the ability to engage in deliberate action. In addition to freedom, other essential qualities of human beings include bonding together with others through human love, the unrestricted desire to know, the appreciation of beauty and goodness, the joy of creative endeavor, the love of God, and the desire for happiness (Banfield, 1997, p. 51).

The object of nursing includes the whole reality of human beings, singly and in social units. This includes individuals, dependent units, and multi-person units such as families and communities.

THE FOUR CONSTITUENT THEORIES
OF SELF-CARE DEFICIT NURSING THEORY

The Theory of Nursing Systems

The nursing system was first conceptualized as a complex action system formed by linking one or a combination of the ways of assisting to a patient self-care system or to some component part of the system (Nursing Development Conference Group, 1973). Nursing systems are designed: (a) to achieve patient health or health-related goals through self-care which is therapeutic, (b) overcome self-care deficits, and (c) foster and preserve self-care abilities of the patient. It establishes the structure and the content of nursing practice. A nursing system is an action system designed by nurses. Inherent in this approach is the position that the nursing system and the self-care system are action systems and that they are open, self-organizing systems, in the sense described by Ashby (1968) and Buckley (1967). These systems have the qualities of conditionality, constraint, and freedom of variation. As open systems become more complex, there develop within them complex mediating processes. These intervene between external forces and behavior and perform the operations of: (1) temporarily adjusting the system to external contingencies; (2) directing the system toward more congenial environments; and (3) permanently reorganizing aspects of the system itself to deal perhaps more effectively with the environment (Backscheider, 1974, p. 1139). The term self, as in "self-regulation," "self-direction," and "self-organizing" points to these mediating processes on the human level.

The power to take action to achieve various goals is known as *agency*. When that power is developed and activated toward care of self it is called *self-care agency*. When it is developed and activated to design and produce nursing systems, it is *nursing agency*. Agency is essential for deliberate action, that is, action that is purposeful, goal directed, thought-out and carried out, or produced. Without question nursing is deliberate action. Nursing agency is developed in nursing education programs, influenced by the many personal, social, cultural, and environmental factors. This agency is refined and further developed through time with reflective experience and additional education. An unreflected experience does little to change nursing agency.

The nursing system was originally conceptualized as a hierarchy of interlocking systems (Orem, 1971, p. 76) as shown in Figure 1.5. This is useful in understanding the many dimensions of nursing situations, the complexity of which should not be underestimated. A nursing situation begins with an interpersonal relationship and interaction within social, contractual, and legal dimensions. The articulations between

FIGURE 1.5   The Science of Self-Care

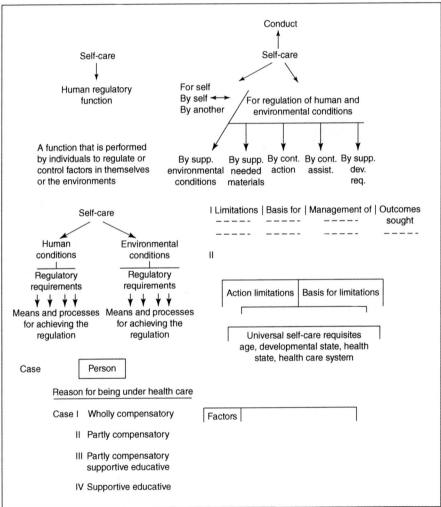

Source: Reprinted from D. E. Orem, 1973, p. 76, with permission of administrator of Orem estate.

self-care, therapeutic self-care demand, and nursing agency constitute the unique nursing aspects of the situation. These ideas are further considered in chapters on nursing practice.

The Theory of Self-Care

The theory of self-care is the second of the constituent theories that form the self-care deficit nursing theory. The concept of self-care was foundational to Orem's work in defining and further developing the self-care deficit nursing theory. The idea of self-care was first used in her 1956 definition and in 1959 description of why persons require and can be helped through nursing. This has been the major focus of theory development and research throughout the years.

The theory of self-care expresses the view of human beings attending to and dealing with themselves. The individual is both the agent of the action (the one acting) and the object of action (the one acted upon). The conceptual elements of the theory are self-care, self-care agency, and self-care requisites. Self-care is an enduring system of actions produced by or for persons from birth to death through the performance of care actions and action sequences. The persons' powers and capabilities for action are referred to collectively as their agency. Self-care agency includes (a) operational powers specific to performing estimative, transitional, and productive result-seeking operations of self-care; and (b) the capabilities and dispositions essential to performing these. The capabilities for self-care are developed over time with assistance and experience in social groups as well as through education and training. Important parts of self-care are self-appraisal and self-management, the effectiveness of which affects the performance of other types of endeavors. Self-care occurs within the broad life situation of the individual, such as family, occupation, education, household, and care and guidance of dependent family members and others. The content related to self-care agency is further developed in Chapter 3.

Self-care requisites are those actions that are required to maintain human functioning and human development and give rise to the development and activation of self-care agency. Requisite refers not just to what is needed for a particular condition, not imposed from the outside (as in required), but is a factor judged necessary according to the nature of things or the circumstances of the case. These requisites may be essential (universal), enduring, or situation specific. The totality of requisites is known as the therapeutic self-care demand. These ideas are developed in Chapter 2.

The Theory of Self-Care Deficit

Deficit expresses a *relationship* between two or more elements where there is not enough resource to meet the essential requisite. It is not a defect in the person's nature or character, though those may be considered in assessing and making judgments about the self-care deficit. In self-care, the essential is identified as the therapeutic self-care demand and the resource as the self-care agency. At any point in time, a person experiences some limitation in ability to meet existing requirements. These may be transitory, short term, easily overcome by gaining information, developing motivation, or seeking assistance. Or the requisites may be more enduring, related to health state or other personal factors including lack of resources. Determination of the nature and extent of the self-care deficit needs to be made before appropriate assistance can be provided. This is an essential part in the development of a nursing system. Nurses may have to use all their skills and knowledge just to diagnose or determine the nature of the self-care deficit, let alone take action working with the person or a designated person, such as a family member, to manage or overcome the deficit. Chapter 4 presents the content of self-care deficit and human assistance.

The Theory of Dependent Care

The theory of dependent care explains how the self-care system is modified when it is directed toward a person who is socially dependent and needs assistance in meeting his or her self-care requisites. This is an area of great interest to many nursing scholars. There are many situations where there are needs for dependent care. In addition to the obvious infant and child care, there are persons with chronic illness or multiple debilitating conditions who are dependent on others for help in meeting self-care requisites. The general structure is analogous to that of self-care. In self-care, the agent and the object are the same individual, whereas in dependent care there are at least two agents only one of whom is the object of the action. This increases the complexity of the situation as it includes capabilities to focus on meeting another's needs and, in many instances, working with the bodily parts of another.

In Chapter 5, dependent-care agency and dependent-care system are examined, as well as the meaning of this for nursing.

SUMMARY

The discipline and profession of nursing are continuing to develop amidst the many changes occurring in the work of health care and higher education, in fact, in the world in general. Within the discipline there is a focus on developing science, philosophy, and other ways of knowing. The profession is concerned about the use of this knowledge to improve patient care through movements such as evidence-based practice. The self-care deficit nursing theory provides a platform for organizing all of these foci and concerns. The self-care deficit nursing theory serves to give direction, meaning, and structure to nursing practice, as well as to emerging theoretic nursing sciences.

REFERENCES

Alligood, M. R., & Tomey, A. M. (2002). *Nursing theory: Utilization and application* (2nd ed.). St. Louis, MO: Mosby.

Argyris, C., Putnam, R., & Smith, D. M. (1985). *Action science*. San Francisco: Jossey-Bass.

Argyris, C., & Schön, D. A. (1974). *Theory in practice: Increasing professional effectiveness*. San Francisco: Jossey-Bass.

Ashby, W. R. (1968). Principles of the self-organizing system. In W. F. Buckley (Ed.), *Modern systems research for the behavioral scientist* (pp. 108–118). Chicago: Aldine Publishing Company.

Banfield, B. E. (1997). *A philosophical inquiry of Orem's self-care deficit nursing theory.* Unpublished doctoral dissertation, Wayne State University, Detroit, MI.

Bekel, G. (1998, February–March). Statements on the object of science: A discussion paper. Paper presented at the meeting of the Orem Study Group, Savannah, GA. *IOS Newsletter, 7*(1999), 11–13.

Buckley, W. (1967). *Sociology and modern systems theory*. Englewood Cliffs, NJ: Prentice-Hall.

Carper, B. A. (1978). Fundamental patterns of knowing in nursing. *Advances in Nursing Science, 1,* 13–23.

Chinn, P. L., & Kramer, M. K. (1999). *Theory and nursing: Integrated knowledge development* (5th ed.). St. Louis, MO: Mosby.

Fawcett, J. (2000). *Analysis and evaluation of contemporary nursing knowledge: Nursing models and theories.* Philadelphia: F. A. Davis Company. Retrieved from EBSCOhost.

Kolcaba, K., & Kolcaba, R. (2011). Integrative theorizing: Linking middle-range nursing theories with the Neuman systems model. In B. Neuman & J. Fawcett (Eds.), *The Neuman systems model.* Boston: Pearson.

Neuman, B., & Fawcett, J. (2011). *The Neuman systems model* (5th ed.). Boston: Pearson.

Nursing Development Conference Group. (1973). In D. E. Orem (Ed.), *Concept formalization in nursing: Process and product.* Boston: Little, Brown. Copyright Orem Estate.

Orem, D. E. (1956). The art of nursing in hospital nursing service: An analysis. In K. M. Renpenning & S. G. Taylor (Eds.), *Self-care theory in nursing: Selected papers of Dorothea Orem.* New York: Springer Publishing Company.

Orem, D. E. (1959). *Guides for developing curricula for the education of practical nurses.* Washington, DC: U.S. Government Printing Office.

Orem, D. E. (1971). *Nursing: Concepts of practice* (1st ed.). New York: McGraw-Hill.

Orem, D. E. (1996). The world of the nurse. In K. M. Renpenning & S. G. Taylor (Eds.), *Self-care theory in nursing: Selected papers of Dorothea Orem* (reprinted 2003, p. 302). New York: Springer Publishing Company.

Orem, D. E. (2001). *Nursing: Concepts of practice* (6th ed.). St. Louis, MO: Mosby.

Paley, J. (2010). Nursing knowledge: Science, practice, and philosophy [Review of the book *Nursing knowledge: Science, practice, and philosophy.* By Mark Risford. Wiley-Blackwell, Oxford]. *Nursing Philosophy, 11*(3), 216–219. ISSN: 1466-7681 PMID: 20536773 CINAHL AN: 2010683449. doi:10.1111/j.1466-769X.2010.00448.x

Renpenning, K. M., & Taylor, S. G. (Eds.). (2003). *Self-care theory in nursing: Selected papers of Dorothea Orem.* New York: Springer.

Schön, D. A. (1983). *The reflective practitioner.* New York: Basic Books.

Sieloff, C. L., & Frey, M. A. (Eds.). (2007). *Middle range theory development using King's conceptual framework* (p. xv). New York: Springer Publishing Company.

Simon, H. A. (1969). *Sciences of the artificial.* Cambridge, MA: The MIT Press.

Smith, M. J., & Liehr, P. R. (2008). *Middle range theory for nursing.* New York: Springer Publishing Company.

Taylor, S. G. (1997). The development of self-care deficit nursing theory: A historical analysis. Paper presented at Sigma Theta Tau conference, Indianapolis, Indiana. *IOS Newsletter* (2nd ed.), 6(November 1998), 7–10.

Weingartner, P. (1976). Wissenschaftstheorie II, 1. Grundlagenprobleme der Logik und Mathematik. Stuttgart: Frommann-Holzboog, Kap 2 and 4.3 [in Bekel, G. (1999, April). Statements of the object of science: A discussion paper. *IOS Newsletter, 7*(1)].

Young, A., Taylor, S. G., & Renpenning, K. (2001). *Connections: Nursing research, theory and practice.* St. Louis, MO: Mosby.

2

The Science of Self-Care

One of the foundational nursing sciences is that of self-care. Increasing the self-care capabilities of persons and communities is of international concern. The rising costs of health care and inadequate numbers of well educated providers is one stimulus for the direction toward self-care. But knowledge of self-care also has the potential for improving the quality of life of individuals, families, and communities. The theory and science of self-care has meaning for anyone and everyone from individuals to policy makers.

Self-care science is a foundational science (Denyes, Orem, Bekel, & SozWiss, 2001) within the structure of the discipline as shown in Figure 1.4 (Chapter 1). Self-care is a complex construct. It is a human regulatory function that one must perform in the interest of life, health, and well-being.

PHILOSOPHIC FOUNDATIONS OF SELF-CARE

The science of self-care begins with knowledge of the human person. Moderate realism and personalism are congruent with the perspective of Self-Care Deficit Nursing Theory (Banfield, 1997; Orem, 2001;

Young, Renpenning, & Taylor, 2001). *Moderate realism* recognizes that a world or reality exists independent of thought and that it is possible to acquire knowledge of this world, recognizing that the reality cannot be fully known. Furthermore, a realist view of reality supports the view that human beings are experiencing beings, beings that attribute meaning based on their experiences and that they have structural and functional differentiations (Banfield, 2001, p. xiv).

Personalism is a philosophy predicated upon the irreducibility and primacy of personal categories, that is, the kind of categories that govern the meaningful interaction among personal beings—"categories of meaning rather than cause, of respect rather than force, of moral value rather than efficacy, of understanding rather than explanation and founded on the fundamental concepts of participation, interpersonal community, and solidarity" (Kohak, 1998). Participation takes place on the "I-Thou" level and entails joining with others. "To participate is to be a co-agent of the community's activities and life, including its self-understanding and self-governance" (Donohue-White, 1997, p. 453).

Nature of Person

The philosophies of realism and personalism affirm both the unique, essentially unrepeatable, and irreducible individuality of the person and the essentially social, relational, contextualized character of the person. "The human is a powerful agent who acts, directly and indirectly, on the substances around him, appropriating them and transforming them in countless ways to suit his needs and desires." (Wallace, 1996, p. 13). The person is "concrete, particular, embodied, living, becoming, developing and being actualized" (Donahue-White, 1997, p. 454). The person is an integrated whole who will never be repeated. Further, that person cannot be reduced to a non-personal being. A person may be the object of study but is not to be treated as an object.

A person is an object in the sense of being subjected to physical forces and able to be acted upon, always keeping in mind that the object is a person with legal and moral standing.

Foundational to self-care deficit nursing theory are the work of Lonergan, Maritain, Harré, and Wallace (Orem, 2001). A more fulsome understanding of the nature of person is essential if one is to make judgments about self-care deficit nursing theory. A common definition of self is that it is the singularity and ultimate uniqueness of every person. The self is the singularity we each feel ourselves to be; it is a site from which a person perceives the world and a place from which to act. The self is the collected attributes of a person, the aspects of a person (Harré, 1998, p. 5). Human beings are "unitary beings who exist in their environment, influencing the world as well as being influenced by the world" (Banfield, 1997, p. 51). A basic knowledge of the self, person, and human being and the differences provides the foundation necessary to grasp the meaning of self-care. Are these distinctions significant or merely "semantics"? Many nurses like to avoid the necessary levels of discourse about such things, preferring to simply dismiss them by saying "it's just semantics" as if words have no distinction or importance. But, in truth, it is much more than semantics, though semantics deals with the meaning of words and is important in communication. When we understand and accept the significance of these concepts, it makes the development of nursing sciences more meaningful and precise. The human can be viewed as a person, agent, user of symbols, unitary human beings or embodied person (organism), and object (NDCG, 1973). As object, the person is subject to physical forces and is the recipient of action. Persons must be able to protect themselves from physical forces, able to control movement and position, know how to act on their own behalf and that of others for whom they are responsible. As users of symbols, persons develop language and ways of communicating, essential to nursing and self-care. Further, the development of nursing science requires a language that provides for inter-subjective meanings and practices that can be shared. It is a matter of knowing rather than feeling, though there is a place for feelings or intuition. In order for nursing to establish itself as a profession and discipline, the words and meanings of the language used needs to be specific to nursing and have agreed upon definitions or meaning, though the language is not necessarily exclusive to nursing.

The embodied person, or organism, refers to the view that human beings are living, functional beings that grow and develop cognitively, psychologically, emotionally, physically, spiritually, and socially throughout the life span. We think of the self as a singular entity and more frequently as a modifier for a multitude of other concepts that describe various aspects of the self as agent or object of action—self-respect, self-consciousness, self-monitoring, self-esteem, and self-care to name but a few.

The agent (person) acts for and upon the self to meet requirements to maintain health and well-being. Health is the state of the living being with respect to their structural and functional wholeness (Orem, 2001). Many parameters of health can be objectively established by comparing existent state with known values. Well-being is the individual's perceived experience of personal life state. It is a subjective evaluation of health state, progress toward personal development, spiritual state, contentment and pleasure. It is possible for a person to be in a poor state of health due to illness, yet have a sense of well-being. Persons with serious disease often describe themselves as having a sense of well-being, a sense that life is good, relationships within the family are good, relationship with God is good, and their overall perception of life is one of well-being. The converse is also possible. Health is explored in more detail in Chapter 4.

Deliberate Action

The science of self-care necessarily includes the ability of the person to act deliberately. This ability or power is referred to as *agency*. Markus and Kitayama (2003) noted that the self is the operational unit and both the source and the locus of control for action. "It is human to act purposefully and to desire to act upon the world. Individual agency, marked by personal attitudinal commitments and a perceived sense of freely choosing to engage in specific behaviors, may be found universally" (Miller, 2003, p. 77).

Human action implies a degree of intrinsic activity. Human action is not strict reactivity to stimuli though there is an element of that inherent in being an organism. Descriptions of deliberate action have a basis in classical philosophy, from Aristotle to more contemporary models and theories. The works of Arnold, Parsons, Wallace, Harré, Gilby, and Macmurray influenced the development of self-care deficit nursing theory (Orem, 2001). Deliberate action refers to actions that have intentions to bring about a particular end or outcome. Self-care, dependent care, and nursing care all require deliberate action. Figure 2.1 presents a model of deliberate action (Orem, 2001, p. 145).

The phases of deliberate action refer to the processes, known as operations. Self-care operations are the processes that are most closely associated with action. Operation is used in the sense of process or action system performed with the goal of meeting self-care requisites. An operation is an intellectual or psychomotor action directed toward a goal or result. Within deliberate action, there are three types of operations: *estimative operations* (to know self-care requisites and means of meeting them), *transitional operations* (to make judgments and decisions about self-care), and *productive operations* (to perform actions to meet self-care demands). The self-care operations are shown above in Table 2.1 (Orem, 2001, pp. 259–260).

FIGURE 2.1   Model of Deliberate Action

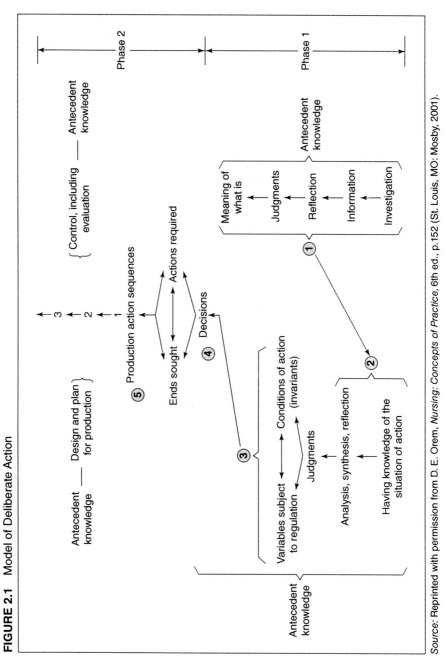

Source: Reprinted with permission from D. E. Orem, *Nursing: Concepts of Practice*, 6th ed., p.152 (St. Louis, MO: Mosby, 2001).

TABLE 2.1
Self-Care Operations

TYPE OF SELF-CARE OPERATION	DESIRED OUTCOME OR GOAL OF OPERATION
Estimative type	
1. Investigation of internal and external conditions and factors significant for self-care	Empirical knowledge of self and environment
2. Investigation of the meaning of characterized conditions and factors and their regulation	Experiential knowing (based in part on acquired technical knowledge) of the meaning of the existent conditions and factors for life, health, and well-being
3. Investigation of the question: How can existent conditions and factors be regulated (i.e., changed or maintained)	Technical knowledge of what can be regulated and the means available for effective regulation
Transitional type	
4. Reflection to determine which course of self-care should be followed	An affirming judgment that one course of self-care is preferred, or that a series of courses is preferred, or that none should be pursued
5. Deciding what to do with respect to self-care	A decision to engage in or not engage in specific regulatory self-care operations
Productive type	
6. Preparation of self, materials, or environmental settings for the performance of a regulatory-type self-care operation	Conditions of readiness for performing self-care operations for regulatory purposes
7a. Performance of productive self-care operations with specific regulatory purposes within a time period	Knowledge that regulatory measures are in process or are completed
7b. Determining presence of and monitoring during performance, of conditions known to affect effectiveness of performance and results	Knowledge that conditions and factors affecting performance and results a. are or are not present b. are or are not under control if present

(Continued)

TABLE 2.1
Self-Care Operations (*Continued*)

TYPE OF SELF-CARE OPERATION	DESIRED OUTCOME OR GOAL OF OPERATION
8. Monitoring for evidence of effects and results a. desired b. untoward	Information about events indicating that regulation is a. being achieved b. not being achieved Knowledge of untoward results a. absence of b. presence of
9. Reflection to determine and confirm evidence of adequacy of performance and presence of regulatory results	An affirming judgment as related to specific self-care regulatory operations a. self-care should continue b. self-care should be discontinued – to be resumed at a specific time – not to be resumed as related to the operations in question
10a. Decision about regulatory operations a. continue action b. close action c. cease action but resume at a specific time	
10b. Decision about estimative operations a. continue to use results obtained from estimative operations (current data base) b. begin a new series of estimative operations	

Source: From Nursing Development Conference Group, Orem D. E. (Ed.), *Concept Formalization in Nursing: Process and Product,* ed. 2, pp. 192–193 (Boston: Little Brown, 1979). With permission of Orem estate administrator.

No one of the three operations can stand in isolation; taking action to meet self-care requisites requires all three operations. The subprocesses of the operations begin with investigation. As listed they are not necessarily sequential; there is movement between and among them. As a person identifies a demand, the process of determining what to do, how to do it, and actually doing it begins with one of the estimative operations, leading to the transitional. As one gathers information or reflects on courses of action, and even begins to take action, that person is likely to need to go back for more information or appraise the situation in order to validate a decision to act. There is little in any of these processes that in reality are linear; there are interaction, feedback loops, reconsiderations, and new information that lead to changes. Ultimately the person must decide and take action, initiating the productive operations. The first phase of action is primarily intellectual. The second phase is that of production of action. As one moves from the first phase to the second, a transition occurs. There is a point at which the person moves from thinking to deciding and beginning to take action. This is known as the transitional operation. These relationships are shown above in Figure 2.1, a model of a general unit of action. All three types of operations are required for deliberate action. The work of gathering knowledge, analyzing and reflecting on this knowledge, making judgments and decision as to actions required to meet desired ends are the estimative and transitional operations. The productive operations are the actions taken to accomplish the end or goal. These operations begin with the command to self that action should begin, activating the powers and capabilities to take action, taking action, evaluating the outcome, and feeling a sense of satisfaction or regret when the action ends. This evaluation frequently triggers another series of action operations leading to the development of an action system (Orem, 2001). Deliberate action is an essential part of self-care and nursing.

There is much that can be said about the nature of person, human agency, and deliberate action. For those interested in the subject, there are hundreds of books available on practically every aspect of human nature and human action. What is necessary is a functional model of person and deliberate action in order to understand Self-Care Deficit Nursing Theory. This is shown in the above Figure 2.1. Further elements are clarified in chapters on the science of self-care, dependent-care, and nursing care.

Persons in Relation

In the previous section, individual, person, and self were identified and described as singular entities. The self is the operational unit in action and is both the source and the locus of control for action. Agency, however, is socially enabled and maintained. All agency is socio-culturally constituted. Markus described the self as both mediator and regulator of behavior,

> [The self] is an organized locus of various understandings of how to be a person, . . . function[ing] as an individualized

orienting, interpreting framework giving shape to what people notice and think about, to what they are motivated to do, to how they feel and their ways of feeling, and to how they act. (Markus, 2003, p. 307)

The construction of the self and agency is "socially mediated and occurs in conjunction with the construction of social relationships" (Markus & Kitayama, 2003, p. 11). When persons are cast as self-directed, they are seen as morally responsible for their action. Persons possess the capacity or the power to act purposively and reflectively and do so in more or less complex relationships with one another. Persons often desire to remake the world in which they live, in circumstances where they may consider different courses of action possible and desirable. Individual agency may be linked with acting on the basis of a perceived sense of what is objectively required or socially expected rather than only with acting in a way that is perceived to be independent of social demands.

Human development is dependent on relationships. Humans live and thrive through a series of interdependent relationships within the primary units of family, community, and culture (Macmurray, 1961). Other persons are the instruments for provision of care, from infancy to maturity, in adult relationships, and in health-related situations. Other persons are considered within the science of self-care as a factor which conditions the requisites for self-care. This is reflected in the self-care requisites, including the maintenance of a balance between solitude and social interaction and the power components of self-care agency. In Orem's words, self-care is the "ability to consistently perform self-care operations, integrating them with relevant aspects of personal, family, and community living" (Orem, 2001, p. 265). Dependent care is, by definition, interpersonal.

Individuals experience themselves as interdependent selves as in relation-to-others, as belonging to social groups, or as significantly and reciprocally enmeshed in families, communities, or work groups. There is agency and there are agents, but these agents do not experience themselves as free from others. The theory of self-care accepts the following constructs:

1. Individual agency is the person who acts and is acted on. "Personal agency allows individuals to realize collective responsibilities while continuing to have a sense of themselves as fully autonomous and free from constraint" (Miller, 2003, p. 82.).

2. Actions involve interdependent selves referencing each other, adjusting to each other, and improving the fit between what one is doing and what is expected. Actions thus require the consideration and anticipation of the perspective of others and are a consequence of the fulfillment of reciprocal obligations or expectations.

3. The inclusion of culture and relationships are basic conditioning factors and foundational capabilities and dispositions that include the concepts of social agency and action.

The content of the *science of self-care* forms the base from which the nursing sciences are developed. Self-care science is viewed as a practical science with both speculative and practical elements drawing from developed nursing science and fields of knowledge as well as from other disciplines. The content areas of the science of self-care include *self-care, self-care requisites and basic conditioning factors, self-care agency with foundational capabilities and dispositions and power components, and self-care deficits* (Orem, 2001). Self-care is the outcome of activated *self-care agency* to meet the *therapeutic self-care demand*.

Key Concepts

■ When the self-care agency (power or capacity to act) is equal to or greater than the demand for action (therapeutic self-care demand), there is no self-care deficit.

■ When the therapeutic self-care demand exceeds the capacity for action, there exists a self-care deficit. The natures of these components of self-care theory are presented later in this chapter and other chapters.

THE THEORY OF SELF-CARE

The essential characteristics of self-care are listed in Exhibit 2.1. The purpose of self-care is to maintain health and well-being and promote development. If persons want to be healthy, grow and develop, they have to take care of themselves. The question that arises is what does one need to do and how does one do it? Self-care is a human regulatory function that one must perform in the interest of life, health, and well-being. The requirements for self-care arise out of the person as unitary

EXHIBIT 2.1
The Characteristics of Self-Care

1. is deliberate,
2. is learned,
3. has purpose,
4. is ego processed,
5. is conduct,
6. is continuous,
7. has pattern and sequence, and
8. has new needs for self-care or to moderate existent self-care actions as a result of injury, illness or disease (Dennis, 1997, p. 37).

human being with all the inner and interpersonal dimensions of self and person within a social and physical environment. A common definition of *self* is that it is the singularity and ultimate uniqueness of each and every person (Harré, 1998, p. 4). There are requisites, actions to be taken, arising out of the universality of persons, the singularity of the self, and the interdependent relationships within the primary units of family and community. The purposes for taking action on behalf of one's self are threefold: to maintain the health and well-being of the person, to provide for continuing development and functioning within norms compatible with conditions essential for life, and to maintain the environment needed to provide for integrated functioning and development. The specifics of these requisites are conditioned by a number of factors, such as age, gender, and health state. Additional conditioning factors include personal relationships within the family, community, culture, and membership in social groups. These factors are referred to as basic conditioning factors and are identified and described further in the chapter.

In self-care, the individual is both the agent of the action (the one acting) and the object of action (the one acted upon). Self-care is deliberate action, in that it is purposeful, involves reflection, judgment, and decision making prior to taking action. Self-care is made up of many discrete actions that over time become an organized whole, referred to as the self-care system. Understanding the self as agent, that is, as one capable of deliberate action, and the self in relation to others is basic to the science of self-care. The theoretical and practical knowledge of self-care expressed in the theory and science of self-care are foundational for both dependent care and nursing care as well as care of self.

Self-care is action directed toward bringing about specific regulation of human functioning and development. There are valid means for meeting these requisites. Further, one must possess the power and capabilities to perform the actions. This regulation of function and development may be met by the self or through the action of another person. This deliberate result-seeking action occurs under existent or changing environmental conditions. The requirement for regulation must be known before effective action can be taken. When identified, formulated and expressed, these requirements and the valid actions for meeting them are known as self-care requisites. The requisites were identified through study of the life sciences, human sciences, and the medical sciences and from the extensive clinical experiences of members of the Nursing Development Conference Group (NDCG).

A cautionary word about the term self-care – much of the literature in many disciplines uses a common sense understanding that focuses on individuals doing things for themselves without specificity. Self-care is also defined as performing activities of daily living with an emphasis on the performance of skills. This is reflected in rehabilitation or long-term care literature. Other literature limits self-care to taking on medical care measures and management of medications. Others believe that critical to the concept of self-care in health is that health-motivated actions initiated by the individual are taken to substitute for or supplement the use of the primary health care system (Fleming, Giachello, Andersen, & Andrade, 1984, pp. 950–951). Self-care is viewed as the primary means for managing symptoms, as a substitute for or supplement to medical care. The self-care deficit nursing theory provides a more holistic perspective and places the focus on the person as individual in maintaining health and well-being throughout life not only in the presence of illness or treatment for disease.

SELF-CARE REQUISITES

The self-care requisites can be established objectively from science. Self-care requisites are products of purposeful investigation of what can and should be regulated. They also include the means that are adequate for regulating specific processes, states, and conditions characteristic of human functioning and development. Self-care requisites are principles to guide the selections, choice, and conduct of regulatory actions in the care of self. The quality and quantity of the requirements are conditioned by certain factors, referred to as basic conditioning factors. Through a process of determining or establishing the conditioning effect of the many factors, the requisite is identified, formulated, and expressed for individuals; this process is referred to as particularizing the self-care requisite. A detailed description of a particularized self-care requisite is presented in Appendix B. Verification of the existence of a self-care requisite is based on empirical and scientific knowledge. Three sets of self-care requisites are identified, namely, universal, developmental, and health deviation.

Universal Self-Care Requisites

Universal self-care requisites are called so because they are common to all human beings and present through all stages of life. They reflect the basic human needs and are essential to maintaining optimum health and well-being. Requisites include the action component necessary to meet the need. It is not enough that a person has a basic need for food; from the perspective of the science of self-care, it is the actions required to meet the need that form the specific focus of attention.

The *universal self-care requisites* are:

1. Maintenance of a sufficient intake of air
2. Maintenance of a sufficient intake of water
3. Maintenance of a sufficient intake of food
4. Provision of care associated with elimination processes and excrements
5. Maintenance of a balance between rest and activity
6. Maintenance of a balance between solitude and social interaction
7. Prevention of hazards to human life, human functioning, and human well-being
8. Promotion of human functioning and development within social groups in accord with human potential, known human limitations, and the human desire to be normal. Normalcy is used in the sense of that which is essentially human and that which is in accord with the genetic and constitutional characteristics and talents of individuals (Orem, 2001, p. 225).

The requisites include both a need for regulatory action and an action component. All persons have a basic human need for water. The amount of fluid needed by a person can be calculated physiologically.

Self-care occurs when the person takes action to maintain the required level of fluid. On a particularly hot day, a person can sometimes tell when there is a need for more fluids by paying attention to his or her bodily functioning such as perspiration, knowing that thirst is not a reliable indicator until dehydration occurs. After appraising the situation, the individual makes the judgment that he or she is fluid depleted and needs to drink more water and change the environment within which he is functioning, such as finding an air conditioned place.

The simple statement of the universal self-care requisite to "maintain an adequate intake of water," does not specify the regulatory results sought; that is, what does adequate mean? The content elements of the requisite can be found in any number of the human sciences. Although that content may be found in disciplines such as sociology, psychology, physiology, and so on, it becomes part of the science of self-care as it is subsumed and interpreted within the essential elements of Self-Care Deficit Nursing Theory. The regulatory results sought and appropriate actions are expressed as part of the science of self-care. The human adult needs approximately 8 hours of sleep per day to maintain health. This requirement for rest varies with the duration and extent of activity. In a test of the effects of different patterns of activity and rest for individuals working in hospitals, doing lifting and other strenuous physical activity, it was found that more frequent, shorter periods of rest were no more recuperative than a single break (Beynon, Burke, Doran, & Nevill, 2000). This kind of study, though not a study within nursing, provides data for understanding the self-care requisite to maintain a balance between rest and activity. The premise of the self-care requisite "maintain a balance between rest and activity" is that both activity and rest are foundational and essential to the life process and actions are needed to bring them into balance. Two underlying self-care requisites essential to meeting this requisite are (a) to maintain a level of physical activity in accord with capabilities and the current standards established for health and well-being, and (b) to obtain a sufficient amount of rest and relaxation to maintain the required and desired level of activity. The literature on activity and rest supports the requisite that maintenance of a balance between activity and rest seeks to control voluntary energy expenditure, regulate environmental stimuli, provide a variety of outlets for persons' interests and talents, and enhance a sense of well-being (Allison, 2007). A balance between activity and rest is necessary to maintain normal bodily rhythms, allow for adaptation, and protect the organism from the excess of rest as immobility and from excessive activity in over stimulation or exertion resulting in wear and tear on all or part(s) of the organism. Selye (1956), in recognizing the need to judiciously balance activity and rest, noted that problems are solved when the mind is in balance and at rest.

The science of self-care includes knowledge of the regulatory requirements and the powers and capabilities to know and meet the requirements. There are also general sets of actions for meeting the eight universal self-care requisites (Orem, 2001, p. 227), as shown in Exhibit 2.2. These general actions provide direction for developing more specific and detailed self-care actions.

EXHIBIT 2.2
General Sets of Actions for Meeting the Eight Universal Self-Care Requisites

1. Maintenance of sufficient intakes of air, water, food
   a. Taking in that quantity required for normal functioning with adjustments for internal and external factors that can affect the requirement or, under conditions of scarcity, adjusting consumption to bring the most advantageous return to integrated functioning
   b. Preserving the integrity of associated anatomic structures and physiologic processes
   c. Enjoying the pleasurable experiences of breathing, drinking, and eating without abuses
2. Provision of care associated with eliminative processes and excrements
   a. Bringing about and maintaining internal and external conditions necessary for the regulation of eliminative processes
   b. Managing the processes of elimination (including protection of the structures and processes involved) and disposal of excrements
   c. Providing subsequent hygienic care of body surfaces and parts
   d. Caring for the environment as needed to maintain sanitary conditions
3. Maintenance of a balance between activity and rest
   a. Selecting activities that stimulate, engage, and keep in balance physical movement, affective responses, intellectual effort, and social interactions
   b. Recognizing and attending to manifestations of need for rest and activity
   c. Using personal capabilities, interests, and values as well as culturally prescribed norms as bases for development of a rest-activity pattern
4. Maintenance of a balance between solitude and social interaction
   a. Maintaining that quality and balance necessary for the development of personal autonomy and enduring social relations that foster effective functioning of individuals

(Continued)

EXHIBIT 2.2
General Sets of Actions for Meeting the Eight Universal Self-Care Requisites
(Continued)

     b. Fostering bonds of affection, love, and friendship, effectively managing impulses to use others for selfish purposes, disregarding their individuality, integrity, and rights
     c. Providing conditions of social warmth and closeness essential for continuing development and adjustment
     d. Promoting both individual autonomy and group membership
  5. Prevention of hazards to life, functioning, and well-being
     a. Being alert to types of hazards that are likely to occur
     b. Taking action to prevent events that may lead to the development of hazardous situations, removing or protecting oneself from hazardous situations when a hazard cannot be eliminated
     c. Controlling hazardous situations to eliminate danger to life or well-being
  6. Promotion of normalcy
     a. Developing and maintaining a realistic self-concept
     b. Taking action to foster specific human developments
     c. Taking action to maintain and promote the integrity of one's human structure and functioning
     d. Identifying and attending to deviations from one's structural and functional norms

Source: From D. E. Orem, *Nursing Concepts of Practice,* 6th ed., p. 227 (St. Louis, MO: Mosby, 2001). With permission of administrator of Orem estate.

There are factors that can condition meeting the universal self-care requisites. These factors are found in the nature, occurrence, or circumstances of a situation that modifies the requirement for action or the ability to perform action and referred to as basic conditioning factors. These are presented later in this chapter.

Developmental Self-Care Requisites

There are three sets of developmental self-care: (1) provision of conditions that promote development, (2) engagement in self-development, and (3) prevention of or overcoming effects of conditions and situations that adversely affect development (Orem, 2001, p. 231). From the science perspective, these are in need of further development and validation in practice. The first of these is met by dependent-care agents in early stages of life. Later in life, it may be the responsibility of others to aid in the provision and maintenance of needed materials and support, for example, in disaster situations or personal illness. The second requires the deliberate involvement of the self in the processes of development. This focuses on developing understanding of and insights about the self through reflection and introspection with a goal of attaining and maintaining positive mental health. The third recognized that there are life events and circumstances that can adversely affect development. For example, becoming paraplegic as an adolescent results in a certain amount of arrested development unless specific measures are instituted to facilitate to prevent that happening.

Health-Deviation Self-Care Requisites

Health-deviation self-care requisites are new and additional requisites arising out of illness or injury and the treatment of such. The changing health state produces requisites related to

1. attending to associated feelings,
2. seeking assistance from appropriate health-care providers,
3. carrying out the recommended actions,
4. attending to the effects of the treatment or care measures, notably those that are discomforting or deleterious,
5. modifying the self by accepting oneself as being in a particular health state in need of treatment,
6. learning to live with the effects of these changed conditions in a life-style that promoted continued personal development and
7. integrating these changes within the family system of living (Orem, 2001, p. 235).

Health deviation self-care requisites are of particular interest to nurses as a large portion of nursing care is performed on behalf of persons experiencing changing health state and needing assistance in managing the associated care measures. In developing the science of self-care, it is useful to consider populations with similar health states. Categories of health-care situations identified by Orem include those oriented to life cycle, recovery from a specific illness or injury, to illness or disorder of undetermined origin, to defects of a genetic or developmental nature and biological immaturity, to active treatment of a disease or disorder (cure or regulation), to restoration, stabilization, or regulation of integrated functioning, when quality of life is gravely affected, and when life cannot continue for long (Orem, 2001, p. 204). General or ideal sets of requisites can be formulated for these health-situations or other populations. These become a part of the data base for particularizing self-care requisites for individuals. These populations or classes of persons with common self-care requisites can be categorized in a number of ways such as by age, by diagnosis, by treatment modality, by response to treatment, or combinations of these. For example, it is possible to generate a set of actions for elderly persons with diabetes, for men with hypertension associated with obesity, persons taking anti-depressant drugs. To have meaning for a specific person, the self-care requisites need to be particularized. The general ideal set of action, first presented by NDCG (1979, p. 282), is presented in Exhibit 2.3. Through years of working with Self-Care Deficit Nursing Theory, this set of actions has proven to be very useful in developing assessment tools, protocols for sets of clients, and managing care for groups of clients. Today, this construct can be useful for nurses developing evidence-based practice protocols. It brings to mind things that need to be considered. For example, the first type of action refers to owning a self with an objectively established state. When a health problem is diagnosed, the person must own it. If the person denies the existence of the problem, they are unlikely to take the prescribed actions and attempts to provide education will not be fruitful. These generalizations are more useful to care agents when the content has been particularized to an individual or a narrowly defined population.

CONDITIONING FACTORS

To take a general statement such as maintain a sufficient intake of food and make it meaningful for the individual is to particularize the requisite. This is done by determining the known or presumed effects of a variety of factors on the form and content of the generalized requisite. These factors are referred to as basic conditioning factors. Formulation of a self-care requisite requires knowledge of human functioning and development under a range of internal and external conditions and requires a thoughtful structuring of facts, concepts, and theories from different sciences and fields of knowledge in articulation with a valid model of deliberate action.

   A number of basic conditioning factors have been identified, including age, gender, developmental state, health state, pattern of living, health care system factors, family system factors, socio-cultural

EXHIBIT 2.3
Diabetes Self-Management

Use this self-care plan:

Nutrition

1. Use your diabetes meal plan. If you do not have one, ask your health care team about one.
2. Make healthy food choices such as fruits and vegetables, fish, lean meats, chicken or turkey without the skin, dry peas or beans, whole grains, and low-fat or skim milk and cheese.
   a. Keep fish and lean meat and poultry portion to about 3 ounces (or the size of a deck of cards).
   b. Bake, broil, or grill it.
   c. Eat foods that have less fat and salt.
   d. Eat foods with more fiber such as whole grains cereals, breads, crackers, rice, or pasta.

Physical activity and tips for maintaining healthy weight:
   Get 30 to 60 minutes of physical activity on most days of the week. Brisk walking is a great way to move more.
   Stay at a healthy weight by using your meal plan and moving more.

General Health:

   a. Ask for help if you feel down. A mental health counselor, support group, member of the clergy, friend, or family member who will listen to your concerns may help you feel better.
   b. Learn strategies to help you cope with stress. Stress can raise your blood glucose (blood sugar). While it is hard to remove stress from your life, you can learn to handle it.
   c. Stop smoking. Ask for help to quit.
   d. Take medicines even when you feel good. Ask your doctor if you need aspirin to prevent a heart attack or stroke. **Tell your doctor if you cannot afford your medicines or if you have any side effects.**
   e. Check your feet every day for cuts, blisters, red spots, and swelling. **Call your health care team right away about any sores that do not go away.**
   f. Brush your teeth and floss every day to avoid problems with your mouth, teeth, or gums
   g. Check your blood glucose (blood sugar). You may want to test it one or more times a day. Use the card at the back of this booklet to keep a record of your blood glucose numbers. **Be sure to take this record to your doctor visits.** Talk with your health care team about your blood glucose targets. Ask how and when to test your blood glucose and how to use the results to manage your diabetes.
   h. Check your blood pressure if your doctor or nurse practitioner advises.
   i. Report any changes in your eyesight to your doctor or nurse practitioner.

Use this plan as a guide to your self-care.
   Discuss how your self-care plan is working for you each time you visit your health care team.

factors, availability of resources, and external environmental factors (Orem, 2001, p. 167). There are relationships between and among conditioning factors (Young, 2001, p. 112). These same factors also condition the self-care agency. The specific values of these factors and their meaning for the individual need to be known before the self-care requisites can be particularized. The values and meaning of the conditioning effect of certain factors are found in other sciences and fields of knowledge. To a great extent the interpretation of values and meaning are found in scientific generalizations and made by a knowledgeable person or health care provider. The list of categories of basic conditioning factors is not all inclusive. It is anticipated that additional factors will be identified; more likely there will be a growing body of knowledge about clusters of basic conditioning factors or interactive basic conditioning factors Figure 2.2.

Moore and Pichler (2000) conducted a review of studies done using basic conditioning factor as a variable. They identified ways in which the basic conditioning factor of family system element was operationally defined and measured. The studies used as operational definitions such things as living arrangement, mother and father's occupation and education, marital status, family expectations, size of family, and social support. They found alternative terms for certain basic conditioning factors and expanded the keywords to include infant, toddler,

FIGURE 2.2   Basic Conditioning Factors

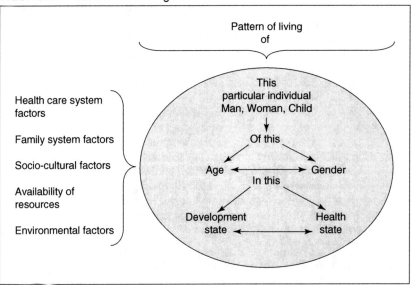

children, school age, high school, adolescent, adult, and elderly (for age); environment (for environmental factors); family (for family system factors); sex (for gender); and socioeconomic status, ethnic, and race (for sociocultural orientation) as they reflect commonly used terminology for these variables. The measurement and interpretation of the values of basic conditioning factors remain a challenge for researchers and practitioners. There is a need to develop more precise categories and subcategories and agreed upon valid measures of these. Although the research supports the theoretical proposition that these basic factors condition the self-care requisite, the way in which this effect occurs is still not known. This is a fertile area for research and theory development.

THE THERAPEUTIC SELF-CARE DEMAND

The *therapeutic self-care demand* is a constructed entity. The components are the particularized self-care requisites including actions and action sequences necessary to meet those requisites. Therapeutic self-care demand refers to *all* of the requisites to be met by or for a person during a specific time period, not just one or two formalized and particularized requisites. Demand implies a level of necessity, urgency, something ignored only with consequences, for example, the increasing intensity of the requisite or exacerbation of the health problem. *Therapeutic* is attached to the term to signify that the processes, actions and action sequences, or care measures for meeting the self-care demand are known or thought to be effective in the situation. For a person to meet the therapeutic self-care demand, the self-care requisites and the actions or processes that need to be taken to meet the requisite must be known. The individual can be helped to know and calculate the therapeutic self-care demand through health education or health promotion activities; the knowledge-base is developed over time and/or in response to a particular health situation. As conditions change, the person may need the assistance of a family member, health-care provider or other knowledgeable person to formulate and express, or calculate, the new or adjusted therapeutic self-care demand. Calculating the therapeutic self-care demand is a search for answers to what series or sequences of action should this person perform in the interests of life, health, and well-being (Orem, 2001).

How does one determine the therapeutic self-care demand? It begins with particularizing each requisite. To do this requires knowledge about the person through the basic conditioning factors—for example, age, gender, family system elements, and health state. Using that data and knowing the science about each, a relationship with the general statement of self-care requisite is established, specifying the value of the regulatory need in both quantity and quality and the associated care actions to meet the need as determined. A 35-year-old American male, single, in a sedentary job, slightly overweight decides to take up bicycle riding this summer. He needs to make some adjustments to his existent self-care system because of the increased activity and his desire to lose weight. The universal self-care requisite to maintain a sufficient intake of water needs to be modified given the increase in activity and the warm environment that will produce increased fluid loss. This universal self-care requisite is conditioned by age in that it is known that healthy sedentary men living in temperate climates should consume 125 oz (3.7 L) of water per day from all dietary sources with about 20% of that coming from dietary sources (Institute of Medicine [IOM], 2004). In addition, amounts of sodium (1.5 g/d), chloride (2.3 g/d), and potassium (4.7 g/d) are needed. The particularized self-care requisite would be to drink at least 125 oz. of fluid each day including at least one bottle of sports drink such as Gatorade. Too much water without the electrolytes can produce hypernatremia. Other self-care requisites that will need modification include maintaining a sufficient intake of food, prevention of hazards, and maintaining a balance between activity and rest. More data would be needed before concluding that other self-care requisites need modification. To maintain cardiovascular health, regardless of weight, adults and children should achieve a total of at least one hour of moderately intense physical activity each day balanced with 7–9 hours of sleep at night. Caloric intake should be 1,800–2,000 per day to lose 1–2 lbs per week. This is best taken equally distributed over three meals with about 200 calories in snacks. He should get 45%–65% of calories from carbohydrates, 20%–35% from fat, and 10%–35% from protein. The recommended intake for total fiber for adults 50 years and younger is set at 38 grams for men (IOM reports, 2002, 2004).

The next step in particularizing the self-care requisite is to the identify methods to be used to meet the requisites. The method to meet the requisite for balance of activity and rest includes bicycle riding while wearing protective gear, or walking for one hour each day. He would need to decide what activities would work for him. He needs to balance this with sleep; though there is no data to suggest a need for change. He could attend to intake by keeping a journal and establishing a dietary plan that includes the IOM recommendations, eating fewer fast foods, cooking nutritional meals. Desired outcomes include weight loss of 20–30 lbs, increased intensity or duration of activity, perceived improvement in well-being, integrating these changes into his overall system of living bringing to the conscious level aspects of self-care that have become habitual, usually as the result of repeated performance.

Once the self-care requisite are particularized, the totality of these and the relationships between and among them needs to be established. This includes the ordering and prioritizing of the requisites considering the immediacy of need and likelihood of accomplishment. In this situation the young man probably needs to place intake of fluids and electrolytes and protection of hazards as priority self-care requisites. The therapeutic self-care demand is usually stated as the collective statements of particularized self-care requisites. In the case of the young man, he may be able to construct his therapeutic self-care demand using his own knowledge and understanding of self and accessing available resources, such as reliable internet sources, nutrition experts in the community perhaps at the local fitness center or grocery store, or in consultation with a health care provider. Through this gaining of information and reflection, the constructed ideal therapeutic self-care demand will be negotiated to one that the person accepts as reasonable and possible. In nursing situations, this is a collaborative process between the nurse and client. This is prescribing the therapeutic self-care demand, that is, making explicit the agreed upon requisites or goals that the person will or must attend to (Orem, 2001). When this step is included, the person is more likely to understand and accept the needs or demands for action that have been identified. A realistic plan for action can then be established that includes consideration of the person's self-care agency. Were the man described in the example to seek assistance from a health care provider, that provider would need to do further assessment generating a more expansive list of factors conditioning his current state of health and well-being. Included in this might be information about his cholesterol and triglyceride level, blood sugar and other physiologic parameters. Perhaps more information about social interactions would be important. Are there family or friends he could exercise with or is the solitude that one has when walking or biking of more importance? What is his usual diet, does he cook and eat at home or in restaurants? The traditional health history and review of systems provides valuable though limited data from self-care and nursing perspectives. *An assessment based in the elements of self-care science from the perspective of self-care deficit nursing theory gives a broader view of the person and current situation.*

The science of self-care includes the science base for each of the self-care requisites and can be found in many disciplines. The content can range from basic hygiene to psychological and physiological influences on the values of the self-care requisite. It includes knowledge of the family system and other social interactions. It explores human development and the influence of age on health and well-being. It includes spiritual life and effects of belief and value systems on interpretation of meaning and value of each self-care requisite. The role of environment on the self-care requisite is another significant conditioning factor. The effects of the Gulf of Mexico oil spill are unknown at this time but are bound to be widespread and difficult to determine at present.

The science of self-care must include new sciences such as that of genomics. As more is learned about how our cells, brain, and body develop and respond based on our genetic makeup, it is likely that there will be changes in our understanding of self-care requisites and human development. It is not likely that the requisite for maintaining an adequate intake of food will change; however, the definitions of adequate and appropriate nutrients are changing. New conceptualizations of the human needs based in a genetic frame of reference could lead to additional requisites or restatements of the content of the existing requisites. One of the features of self-care deficit nursing theory is that it provides a framework for integrating new knowledge into the existing framework, making the knowledge available for use in practice.

An example of this is the incorporation of genetics into a revision of the structure of Maslow's basic human needs theory, developed by Yang (2003), with three categories of needs: genetic survival, genetic transmission, and genetic expression (p. 227). Yang proposes that given the considerably instinctual nature of basic human needs, a better way to choose and categorize them may be the application of some general concepts in human genetics. One set of such concepts is genetic survival (keeping one's genes alive by keeping oneself alive), genetic transmission (passing on one's genes to offspring), and genetic expression (realizing the personal potentials given by one's genes during one's own life span). From the evolutionary point of view, there are two basic adaptive problems for any organism, namely, individual survival and reproduction, with the former essentially subsidiary to the latter. For human beings, however, individual survival is the common prerequisite for genetic survival, which in turn is the precondition for genetic transmission and expression. Of these, Yang postulates that genetic survival and genetic transmission are universal, but genetic expression is variable and culture-bound. Arranged on the stem of the Y are Maslow's physiological needs (excluding sexual needs) and safety needs. Satisfaction of these needs is indispensable to genetic survival. On the stem of the Y, are the two categories or levels of needs that, if well satisfied, guarantee the organism's biological existence, which in turn guarantees the physiological survival of the organism's genes. On the left arms of the Y are interpersonal and belongingness needs, esteem needs, and the self-actualization need for individuals and collectivities. The thoughts and behaviors required for the fulfillment of these needs lead to genetic expression. Lastly, on the right arm of the Y are sexual needs, childbearing needs, and parenting needs; the five categories of needs that fulfill reproductive functions and lead to the intergenerational transmission (duplication) of the organism's genes (Yang, 2003). The thoughts and behaviors entailed in the satisfaction of these needs result in genetic transmission. If this model has validity, and there is considerable literature that supports this, what does it mean to the theory of self-care and to the work of self-care scientists? Might there be need for modifications in the universal and/or developmental self-care requisites? The needs on both the right and left arms of the Y could be construed as developmental requisites. Or perhaps there needs to be a reconstruction of the requisite for normalcy within the self-care deficit nursing theory.

SELF-CARE PRACTICES AND SELF-CARE SYSTEMS

The proper object or reality focus of the science of self-care is the person in human societies continuously producing systems of self-care. *A self-care system* is comprised of performed actions and sequences of actions by persons to regulate their functioning and development in concrete life situations. *Self-care practices* and systems are evidence of the person's engagement in self-care. These systems are largely generated through habit, or customary use, an acquired behavior pattern that is almost involuntary, except when there are changes in requisites or environmental conditions or when the performance of the habit deteriorates to the point that it is no longer effective. A practice becomes habitual through repetitive performance. Initially there is deliberate thought, intention to act, action, and evaluation of performance. Self-care systems are made up of skillful actions. The features of skillful action are that it is effective, it appears to be effortless, and the actor need not think about how to do it (Argyris & Schön, 1974, p. 50). *Self-care actions* are the components of the self-care system; the actions sequences are performed during the production phase of self-care and the effects of the actions endure over time. Self-care systems reflect the known therapeutic self-care demand and the actions the person is able and willing to perform at the time the system is being produced. The concept of system is helpful to this discussion. There are two characteristics of note. The first is the premise that the whole is greater than and different from the sum of the parts. The second premise is that the elements or parts of the system work together as a whole; hence, a change in one part affects the whole (Geden & Taylor, 1999). As noted in Chapter 1, self-care systems are action systems that are open, self-organizing systems with the qualities of conditionality, constraint, and freedom of variation. Changes in the therapeutic self-care demand lead persons to (1) temporarily adjust the self-care system to external contingencies, (2) direct the system toward more congenial environments, and (3) permanently reorganize aspects of the system itself.

Self-care systems occur within broader systems of living of the person but there is interaction among the self-care system and other systems, such as financial. As a writer, my broader system of living involves sitting at the computer, organizing thoughts and words, sometimes stopping to play with my dog attending to her needs. The aspects of my self-care system intersect with the work system. I know that I need to get up to attend to self-care requisites for sufficient food and water, and processes of elimination. I accept that I have an imbalance between solitude and social interaction but this is temporary. I need to watch my posture and do exercises, like flexing my feet and knees to prevent hazards. I take my dog for a walk to get more exercise, improving the balance between rest and activity. Later, I'll turn on Wii® and do some aerobic exercises, stretching, and balance activities. I also know that not all actions taken to meet requisites are therapeutic; some in fact may be harmful. I don't eat enough leafy green vegetables; I eat more carbohydrates than I should. Obesity is epidemic in the United States. Other persons smoke cigarettes. It is hard to imagine that there are people in our society who don't know the dangers of smoking. These self-care actions or behaviors are not therapeutic in outcome. However, there are many persons who don't understand the dangerous effects of smoking or being overweight or don't have the knowledge or support to change these behaviors. Action is required at the social level as well as the personal level to effect healthier behaviors.

Self-care practices are anything but natural acts; they are cultur-ally saturated processes that entail engagement with culture-specific sets of meanings and practices. Social psychologists are well aware that the construction of the self and agency is socially mediated and occurs in conjunction with the construction of social relationships. In Figure 2.3 Yang (2003) has shown a model that conjoins the collective

FIGURE 2.3   Double Y Model of Basic Human Needs

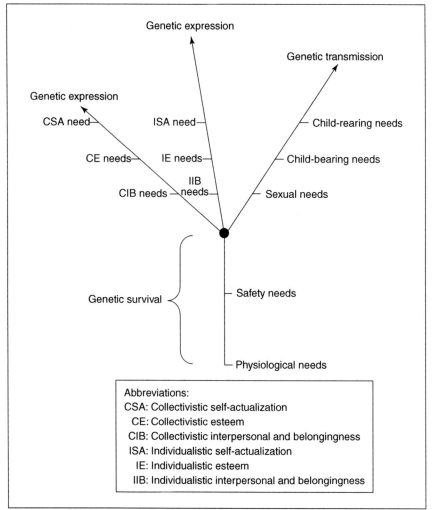

Source: Reproduced from *Cross-Cultural Differences in Perspectives on the Self,* Vol. 49 of the Nebraska Symposium on Motivation by permission of the University of Nebraska Press. Copyright 2003 by the University of Nebraska Press.

and individual approaches to basic needs. Incorporation of this model into our understanding of basic needs as well as extending our thinking to genetics provides a cross-cultural perspective. The needs are congruent but the manner of meeting the needs varies from individualistic to collectivistic cultures, conditioning the self-care practices of persons.

SELF-CARE BEHAVIORS, SELF-MANAGEMENT

There are a number of measures performed by the person that can be called *self-care behaviors*. These are externally and internally oriented actions. The results of the operations of deliberate action – estimative, transitional, and productive – are the basis for understanding self-care behaviors. These include a focus on persons in physical environments, in social environments with given roles and role expectations, and a personal frame focused on personal values, the self-as-felt and known, the ideal self, and long-range goal orientations. Internally oriented self-care actions are resource-using action sequences to control internal factors and action sequences to control oneself (thoughts, feelings, orientation) and thereby regulate internal factors or one's external orientations (Orem, 2001, p. 269). Internally oriented self-care behaviors at any particular time depend in part on acquired knowledge about the goals and practices of self-care including knowledge about the nature and meaning of self-care, in self-care skills, and in initiating, directing, and controlling behavior to accomplish defined goals of self-care. Externally oriented self-care behaviors are need-fulfilling behaviors with an external environmental orientation. These include:

- knowledge-seeking action sequences,
- assistance- and resources-seeking action sequences,
- expressive interpersonal actions,
- action sequences to control external factors (Orem, 2001, p. 269)

Performed self-care measures become the system of self-care, sometimes requiring modifications, major or minor. The controlling of the system or various aspects of the system is called *self-management*. This is a term used extensively in the pharmacology literature to describe the actions needed to manage a particular medication within a particular illness, for example, self-management of diabetes using insulin.

Within the science of self-care, self-management refers to controlling, handling, directing, or governing the actions in a particular environment at a particular time. These executive abilities, like other self-care actions, need to be developed and deliberately produced. Critical elements of self-management within or about the self-care system need explication and explanation. In certain health-situations, there are standardized models for self-management. Diabetes is a good example. Sousa (2003) present a model of self-management that includes self-care deficit nursing theory. The National Institute of Diabetes and Digestive and Kidney Diseases (NIDDK) has developed a self-care plan or self-management plan 2009. These actions are a part of the self-care system of a person with type 2 diabetes. These actions need to be integrated in the broader systems of self-care and daily living. These are presented in Exhibit 2.3, Diabetes Self-Management.

SUMMARY

The science of self-care is an ever expanding field of knowledge. The knowledge is not exclusive to nursing. Though it is developed and used in many fields of science and practice, it is the basis for the self-care deficit nursing theory. How persons care for themselves and others for the purpose of maintaining health and well-being through meeting the requirements for self-care is basic to understanding the persons' limitations for action. The next chapter will explore the ways in which persons are able to act on their own behalf or for others.

REFERENCES

Allison, S. E. (2007). Self-care requirements for activity and rest: An orem nursing focus. *Nursing Science Quarterly, 20*, 68.

Argyris, C., & Schön, D. A. (1974). *Theory in practice: Increasing professional effectiveness.* San Francisco: Jossey-Bass.

Banfield, B. E. (1997). *A philosophical inquiry of Orem's self-care deficit nursing theory.* Unpublished doctoral dissertation, Wayne State University. ProQuest AAT 9815271; OCLC/World Cat No. 39737970.

Banfield, B. E. (2001). Philosophical foundations of Orem's work. In D. E. Orem (Ed.), *Nursing: Concepts of practice* (6th ed., pp. xi–xvi). St. Louis, MO: Mosby.

Beynon, C., Burke, J., Doran, D., & Nevill, A. (2000). Effects of activity–rest schedules on physiological strain and spinal load in hospital-based porters. *Ergonomics, 43*(10), 1763–1770.

Dennis, C. (1997). *Self-care deficit theory of nursing: Concepts and applications* St. Louis, MO: Mosby.

Denyes, M. J., Orem, D. E., & SozWiss, B. G. (2001). Self-care: A foundational science. *Nursing Science Quarterly, 14*(1), 48–54.

Donohue-White, P. (1997) Understanding equality and difference: A personalist proposal. *International Philosophical Quarterly, 37*(4), 441–456.

Fleming, G. V., Giachello, A. L., Andersen, R. M., & Andrade, P. (1984). Self-care: Substitute, supplement, or stimulus for formal medical care services? *Medical Care, 22*(10),

Geden, E., & Taylor, S. (1999). Theoretical and empirical description of adult couples' collaborative self-care systems. *Nursing Science Quarterly, 12,* 329–334.

Harré, R. (1998). *The singular self: An introduction to the psychology of personhood.* Thousand Oaks, CA: Sage.

Institute of Medicine of the National Academies. (2002, September 5). *Dietary reference intakes for energy, carbohydrate, fiber, fat, fatty acids, cholesterol, protein, and amino acids report.* Retrieved from the http://www.Iom.Edu/Reports/2002/Dietary-Reference-Intakes-For-Energy-Carbohydrate-Fiber-Fat-Fatty-Acids-Cholesterol-Protein-And-Amino-Acids.aspx

Institute of Medicine of the National Academies. (2004, February 11). *Dietary reference intakes: Water, potassium, sodium, chloride, and sulfate consensus report.* Retrieved from http://www.iom.edu/Reports/2004/Dietary-Reference-Intakes-Water-Potassium-Sodium-Chloride-and-Sulfate.aspx

Kohak, E. (1998). *Personalism: A brief account.* Retrieved from http://www.philosophy.ucf.edu/pi/pers.html

Macmurray, J. (1961). *Persons in relation.* New York: Harper and Brothers.

Markus, H. R. (2003). Epilogue: A conversation. In V. Murphy-Berman & J. Berman (Eds.), Cross-cultural differences in perspectives on the self. *Cross-cultural differences in perspectives on the self (eBook): Current theory and research in motivation* (Vol. 49). Lincoln, NE: University of Nebraska Press.

Markus, H. R., & Kitayama, S. (2003). Models of agency: Social diversity in the construction of action. In V. Murphy-Berman & J. Berman (Eds.), *Cross-cultural differences in perspectives on the self (eBook): Current theory and research in motivation* (Vol. 49). Lincoln, NE: University of Nebraska Press.

Miller, J. G. (2003). Culture and agency: Implications for psychological theories of motivation and social development. In V. Murphy-Berman & J. Berman (Eds.), *Cross-cultural differences in perspectives on the self (eBook): Current theory and research in motivation* (Vol. 49). Lincoln, NE: University of Nebraska Press.

Moore J. B., & Pichler, V. H. (2000). Measurement of Orem's basic conditioning factors: A review of published research. *Nursing Science Quarterly, 13*(2), 137–142.

NDCG. (1973). *Concept formalization in nursing: Process and product.* Orem, D. E. (Ed.). Boston: Little Brown.

NDCG. (1979). *Concept formalization in nursing: Process and product* (2nd ed.). Orem, D. E. (Ed.). Boston: Little Brown.

National Institute of Diabetes and Digestive and Kidney Diseases. (2009). *4 steps to control your diabetes. For life* (Publication No.NDEP-67).

Orem, D. E. (2001). *Nursing: Concepts of practice* (6th ed.). St. Louis, MO: Mosby.

Selye, H. (1956), *The stress of life.* New York: McGraw-Hill.

Sousa, V. D. (2003). Testing a conceptual framework for diabetes self-care management (Doctoral dissertation. Case Western Reserve University, 2003). *Dissertation Abstract International, 64,* 3193.

Sousa, V. D., Zauszniewski, J. A., Musil, C. M., McDonald, P. E., & Milligan, S. E. (2004). Testing a conceptual framework for diabetes self-care management. *Research and Theory for Nursing Practice: An International Journal, 18*(4), 293–316.

Wallace, W. A. (1996). *The modeling of nature: Philosophy of science and philosophy of nature in synthesis.* Washington, DC: The Catholic University of America Press.

Yang, Kuo-Shu. (2003). Beyond Maslow's culture bound linear theory: A preliminary statement of the double-Y model of basic human needs. In V. Murphy-Berman & J. J. Berman (Eds.), *Cross-cultural differences in perspectives on the self: Current theory and research in motivation* (Vol. 49). Lincoln, NE: University of Nebraska Press.

3

The Science of the Development
and Exercise of Self-Care Agency

W hat knowledge and skills need to be put into action to meet the demands for self-care described in the preceding chapter? And what if the person is unable to meet those demands? That which enables a person to accomplish the work of self-care is referred to as *self-care agency*. Self-care agency is the power of the person to engage in self-care behaviors; the results or product of the use of those powers are self-care actions and the system of self-care. The broad structure of self-care agency is modeled on the structure of deliberate action presented in Chapter 2, Figure 2.1. Self-care agency is a mechanism for determining the components of the therapeutic self-care demand as well as a means for accomplishing the required care. The therapeutic self-care demand sets the specifications for the self-care agency needed in a particular situation. When the self-care agency is not adequate, some components of the therapeutic self-care demand will not be met; this deficit relationship between demand and agency is a *self-care deficit*.

The *science of the development and exercise of self-care agency* is a subset of the science of self-care. While agency, the power to act or the potential for action, is an attribute of being human, self-care agency is a particular type of power: the power or potential to take care of the self in matters of health. Self-care agency must also be distinguished from other forms of agency, for example, moral agency which is the power or capacity to make choices regarding right and wrong. Ways of caring for one's self, of promoting mental and physical development and health, are not inborn; they must be learned. Self-care agency must be developed. Self-care requires that a person use memory, imagination, and reasoning, make judgments and decisions, and perform tasks. When there are situations or conditions that limit the person's action capabilities to gain knowledge, make judgments and decisions or take action, there exists a self-care deficit. All persons experience self-care deficits at different times and in different ways. A self-care deficit exists when the person's self-care agency is not sufficient to meet the on-going therapeutic self-care demand. A self-care deficit states a *relationship* between the therapeutic self-care demand and self-care agency. The person's awareness of some aspect of a self-care deficit, some self-care limitation, is the stimulus for action on his or her own behalf or for seeking assistance. When these limitations are related or articulated with a particularized requisite, it describes a self-care deficit or a component of a self-care deficit. The essential element of *self-care deficit nursing theory* is the presence of a health-associated self-care deficit that establishes a need for, and gives direction to, nursing.

SELF-CARE AGENCY

The reality focus or *proper object* of the science of self-care agency is the *"human powers activated and evidenced by persons when they perform the investigative, judgment, decision-making, and productive operations of self-care"* (Orem, 2001, p. 178). Self-care, considered as self-initiated, self-directed, and self-permitted behavior, will be engaged only when the person is in a state which allows for the voluntary regulation and direction of behavior toward defined goals of self-care. Self-care agency in the mature adult is generally anticipated to be adequate to meet the therapeutic self-care demand.

One of the attributes of people is that they have the capacity for forethought. This enables them to organize and regulate their lives proactively. Human self-regulation occurs when the persons motivate and guide their actions through proactive control by setting themselves valued goals, mobilizing their abilities and efforts based on what they expect is required to reach the goals. Feedback control comes into play in subsequent adjustments of strategies and effort to attain desired results. After people attain the goal they have been pursuing, those with a strong sense of self-efficacy set higher goals for themselves. Self-efficacy is one of the foundational dispositions for self-care agency. Development of the self-care system follows a similar pattern through the self-care operations. A thoughtful plan for future deliberate action is called intention.

Prior to deliberate action, the agent intellectually develops ideas about what needs to be accomplished and decides which actions ought to be taken. Knowledge is derived from experiences as one plans action, takes action, and then reflects on the results achieved. As new knowledge is gained from each situation, more choices or alternatives become evident. With trial and error experiences and assistance in interpreting the outcomes, agents learn to make a selection among possible (known) action sequences. Eventually, from the newly formed knowledge base, one approach is selected as the best approach and, with practice, a patterned action sequence, or habits, results (Cox & Taylor, 2005, p. 250).

Self-care agency needs to be developed, operative, and activated if care is to be produced. Self-care requires both learning and the use of knowledge as well as motivation and skill. The model of deliberate action, Figure 2.1 indicates the importance of antecedent knowledge to the self-care operations by bracketing the estimative, transitional, and productive operations. The way a person investigates a situation, gives it meaning, considers actions to be taken, and finally takes action and evaluates the results are limited by the person's repertoire of knowledge and skills. Early on in the process and at various points in the process, the person might recognize a need for additional knowledge. The awareness of the need for knowledge and the knowledge-seeking skills of the person will give direction to the action taken. Some persons ask older family members or friends, some seek out their own information on the Web or in a library, whereas others seek assistance from health-care professionals. Health-seeking behaviors and health promotion research provide useful information in looking at ways in which self-care agency may be conditioned. There is a need for more research to specifically demonstrate this.

The structure of self-care agency includes foundational capabilities and dispositions for action, power components for self-care, and self-care operations. In addition to the capabilities for performing estimative, transitional, and productive self-care operations, there are the power components that enable performance of these operations, and the foundational capabilities and dispositions that set the parameters

FIGURE 3.1   The Structure of Self-Care Agency

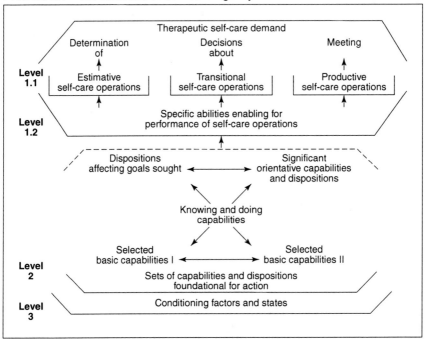

Source: Reprinted with permission from NDCG, *Concept Formalization in Nursing: Process and Product,* p. 230 (Boston: Little, Brown, 1979).

within which the power components can operate. Figure 3.1 depicts these relationships.

Although there are many powers and capabilities for deliberate action in general, those necessary for self-care action are specific to self-care. For example, the identified estimative operations are particular to investigating factors significant for self-care and deciding what to do in respect to self-care. The power components are directly related to self-care as they specify the particular power the person needs to have developed to perform the self-care operations, for example, the ability to reason is specific to reasoning within a self-care frame of reference. The human capabilities and dispositions are identified as being foundational for self-care agency. Knowledge of these conditioning factors and power component come from other sciences as well as nursing science and research. The value and meaning of these factors are articulated and validated within theories of self-care and self-care agency to become part of the foundational nursing sciences.

SELF-CARE OPERATIONS

Self-care operations are the processes used to perform self-care. These are identified in three sets referred to as the estimative, transitional, and productive operations. Estimative operations refer to investigative processes, whereas transitional operations refer to processes of judgment and decision making. Productive operations are the processes necessary to perform action. These are detailed below.

Phase 1: Estimative and Transitional Self-Care Operations

The estimative and transitional operations were first described by the NDCG and presented in *Concept Formalization in Nursing*, 2nd edition, 1979. Orem continued to use them unchanged in her latest writing. The operations and the results of activating them are shown in Table 2.1 (see Chapter 2). The transitional operations end with a commitment to take action. The productive operations begin with the preparation of self and materials concluding with reflection/evaluation of the results and decisions concerning continued action.

Phase 2: Productive Self-Care Operations

The productive operations are necessary to perform actions to meet self-care requisites. They include cognitive processes as well as the psychomotor skills needed for performance of actions. The productive self-care operations are shown in Table 2.1.

Having determined the regulatory goals to be achieved, that is, therapeutic self-care demand, and the specific operations that need to be performed, the next concern is the person's ability to perform these actions. The power necessary to the development and exercise of self-care operations is the next substructure of self-care agency.

POWER COMPONENTS OF SELF-CARE AGENCY

The power components are intermediate between operations and the foundational capabilities and dispositions. Ten power components were identified and are presented in Exhibit 3.1.

These power components, intermediate with self-care operations and foundational capabilities and dispositions necessarily articulate

EXHIBIT 3.1
Foundational Capabilities and Dispositions

A survey list of human capabilities and dispositions foundational
to the human power, self-care agency, with a list of conditioning
factors and states.

Conditioning Factors and States
    Genetic and constitutional factors
    Arousal state
    Social organization
    Culture
    Experience
Capabilities and Dispositions
    Selected basic capabilities
        Sensation
            Proprioception
            Exteroception
        Learning
        Exercise or work
        Regulation of the position and movement of the body and its parts
        Attention
        Perception
        Memory
        Central regulation of motivational and emotional processes
    Knowing and doing capabilities
        Rational agency
        Operational knowing
        Learned skills
            Reading, counting, writing
            Verbal, perceptual, manual
            Reasoning
        Self-consistency in knowing and doing
    Dispositions affecting goals sought
        Self-understanding, self-awareness, self-image
        Self-value, self-acceptance, self-concern
        Acceptance of bodily functions
        Willingness to meet needs of self
        Future directedness
    Significant orientative capabilities and dispositions
        Orientations to time, health, other persons, events and objects
        Priority system or value hierarchy
            moral, economic, aesthetic, material, social
        Interests and concerns
        Habits
        Ability to work with the body and its parts
        Ability to manage self and personal affairs

Source: Reprinted from NDCG, *Concept Formalization in Nursing: Process and Product,* p. 212 (Boston: Little, Brown, 1979). Used with permission of Walene E. Shields, heir of Dorothea E. Orem.

with one or more of the self-care operations. The "ability to control the positions of the body and its parts" is not necessarily associated with the transitional operations of making judgments and decisions about self-care or with the productive operations of reflection and decisions but it is essential for doing the actions. This becomes important in the wholly and partly compensatory nursing sciences (Chapter 8). Not all the associations are of equal significance; some are necessary but not critical. For example, the power component "maintain attention and requisite vigilance," while necessary for all operations, is critical for operations to acquire empirical and technical knowledge. These components are unchanged since first published in 1979 and "are in need of refinement and further development in respect to their own structure and to their articulations with self-care operations and foundational capabilities and dispositions" (Orem, 2001, p. 264).

FOUNDATIONAL CAPABILITIES AND DISPOSITIONS

As described, persons have powers of action. Underlying these powers are human capabilities and dispositions. "Dispositions are observable properties of individuals, the predominant or prevailing tendency of one's spirit" (Harré, 1998, p. 117). "Dispositions, understood as tendencies to behave in certain ways in certain situations include desires, beliefs, attitudes, abilities and psychological traits" (Argyris & Schön, 1974, p. 55). In self-care deficit nursing theory, dispositions refer to conditions that affect persons' willingness to look at themselves and accept themselves as self-care agents, to accept themselves as in need of particular self-care measures or to perform certain self-care measures (Orem, 2001). Self-understanding, self-concern, self-image, self-efficacy all affect a person's willingness to perform self-care measures and the ways in which he/she will process information and make decisions about action. If someone faints at the sight of blood, he or she probably won't be disposed to perform self-care measures when injured.

Capabilities basic to human action which can be used or developed are essential for engagement in self-care. The level of the capability or the capacity for something may set limits on the persons' ability to develop, exercise, or activate the power components and self-care operations. If someone doesn't have the capability to move the body and its parts, he or she will be limited in what kind of measures can be taken. On the other hand, limited capacity for movement need not limit the learning capacity or decision-making ability. The human capabilities and dispositions foundational for self-care are shown in Exhibit 3.1.

Variations in the development, exercise, and operability of self-care agency originate in the foundational capabilities and dispositions. If a person has a memory impairment, there may be limitations in the development of self-care agency. The person may not remember or recall things previously learned, such as certain skills or the antecedent knowledge needed for decision-making. There may be limitations in the ability to learn new self-care measures. It may require much repetition of an action before the skill is developed and retained so it can be used or exercised appropriately. When assessing self-care agency, it is necessary to recognize that the basic factors may be conditioning the power components and the capability to carry out the required self-care operations. The articulation between foundational capabilities and dispositions and a basic conditioning factor of altered health state associated with cognitive disorders can mean that the foundational capabilities and dispositions of operational knowing are affected. Operative knowing and its states are used in the sense defined by Inhelder and Piaget (1958). His *theory of cognitive development* focuses on the development of the intellect within four major periods of cognitive development: sensorimotor, preoperational thought, concrete operations, and formal operations. If the level of knowing is only at the concrete operational level, the ways in which information about self-care measures is presented needs to be at a level that can be comprehended and made operational.

The translation of requirements for action into action calls for the coordination of specific human capabilities. Absence of a portion of these capabilities results in a limitation in meeting these requirements. Reporting on the work at the Diabetic Nurse Management Clinic at Johns Hopkins Center, Backscheider (1974) described the foundational capabilities essential to therapeutic self-care for diabetes, moving from the general capability to the specific capability needed for identified aspects of the regimen for therapeutic self-care of diabetes. These concepts apply to anyone needing to develop a complex system of self-care for themselves or assisting others (see Chapter 7).

Since the initial development by the NDCG, there has been amplification in understanding the underlying concepts of self-care agency; amplification because the original definition and concept have not changed. This amplification continues today and needs to continue and be integrated into the science of self-care. Significant development occurred and was reported in the 2nd edition of *Concept Formalization in Nursing* (1979) and by Orem in all six editions of *Nursing: Concepts of Practice*. Many scholars, researchers, and practitioners contribute to our understanding of self-care. Knowledge about self-care agency is essential for identifying and understanding the nursing sciences and nursing practice, presented in Section II.

Taking self-care measures assumes that self-care agency is developed and that it can be activated or exercised. There is much that a person knows about appropriate self-care measures to meet emerging self-care demands. For most people self-care agency is developed so that on a sunny summer day, they know actions they need to take to prevent serious sunburn or heat stroke. But those measures won't be taken if the person doesn't activate the self-care agency and initiate the actions. If one goes out unprotected, the actions are not therapeutic and the results will be harmful. So though self-care agency may be developed through health teaching, it is adequate only if it also deals with issues of resources, values and motivation, for example. Having a tan is considered a beauty enhancement within a sector of U.S. culture; for some persons, especially young adult white women, beauty is a higher value than self-care and they fail to exercise their self-care agency by choosing inappropriate food intake. The same language and examples cannot be used for a child as an adult. Backscheider (1974) estimated that in the Diabetic Nurse Management Clinic, about 30% of the patients could not read. That factor necessitated the design of a system wherein much of the information and teaching was exchanged through verbal contact and not literature. When so much information exchange relies on reading, such as on the web, persons are even more disenfranchised.

DEVELOPMENT OF SELF-CARE AGENCY

The ability to perform self-care is conditioned by levels of development. Parents initiate and direct systems of infant and child care and help the child gradually develop a system of self-care. One significant source from which a person learns about self-care and self-care practices is culture, that is, the beliefs and habits that characterize the way of living of a group of people. The individual for the most part learns of the culture's standards within the family. In American culture, in addition to the family, and sometimes in place of them, peers, the school, radio and television, Internet, and health professionals are sources of information regarding self-care.

Development viewed from the sciences of the human development forms the basis for understanding the stages of development and the assumptions about the development of self-care agency. The process of development of self-care agency from infancy to adulthood is not well documented. Many studies focus on the self-care practices of children with specific health-related needs, such as diabetes and asthma (Cox & Taylor, 2005; Moore & Beckwith, 2006). At some time the results of these studies need to be consolidated into a theory of the development of self-care agency by age, stage of human development, and health state. Other conditioning factors such as culture and family should also be integrated. Early on in life there is a correlation between the parent/responsible person's self-care agency and the developing child's self-care agency.

Children have to learn about self-care and develop the ability to accomplish self-care. Ways of caring for oneself are not inborn; infants and children do not innately possess self-care agency. They do have the potency or potential for developing self-care agency within the context of foundational capabilities and dispositions and basic conditioning factors. The process begins when the infant responds instinctually; over time these instinctive responses become habituated and more complex in response to the care giver. The person learns about self-care in the family and culture. Each individual develops his or her own system of self-care within a larger system or way of living. Thus self-care practices may affect or be affected by other aspects of daily living as well as by the physical and social environment in which a person lives. The person can only be a mature self-care agent when the person has reached that stage of development which permits him or her to knowingly direct and control his/her behavior to achieve specific results. Parents and others initiate and direct systems of infant and child care and help the child gradually develop his/her own system of self-care. The developing self-care system augmented by input from adults and peers changes as the child moves into adolescence and then adulthood, finally becoming the person's own self-care system. It is significant that "human beings are never completely self-sufficient; they come into the world dependent on parents, grow up within a family context, and require the additional resources of city or state to reach intellectual and moral maturity" (Wallace, 1996, p. 187).

One example of the effect of growing up in traditional U.S. culture, where women are viewed as the primary caregiver is described by Low (1993) as she talks about caring for her mother who has a chronic disease.

"The myth of nurturing or caring as exclusive to women not only obscures the processes by which women become care givers, it also obscures the processes by which men learn or do not learn to care . . . caring taken on by men like my father and brother is 'viewed as exceptional' as it does not conform to traditional patterns of caring. I see my brother and father not so much as exceptions, but as examples of the potential elasticity of gender roles. For lack of a more appropriate concept, I have seen the 'feminization' of my father and brother, their rapid socialization into care givers. Future research would do well to examine how men learn to care." (Low, 1993, p. 39)

Gender differences in the development of self-care agency also need to be explicated. What contributions do fathers make to the development of self-care agency for sons, daughters? Are they different between sons and daughters? And mothers? Do children of single parents of either gender develop self-care agency in similar ways; do they experience differences in self-care capabilities or limitations in self-care abilities? Are gender differences only cultural or are there other ways in which gender conditions the development and operability of self-care agency?

At each developmental stage, children are capable of certain self-care actions, and as their self-care agency increases, parental assistance decreases. Fan (2008) noted that the school-age period is usually the first time that children begin to make truly independent judgments. School age children are interested and able to contribute to their own health history. A sense of industry normally develops during the ages of 6–12 years. With the sense of autonomy and initiative in place, the child is ready to engage in tasks that can and will be followed through to completion. They are interested in learning and mastering new skills and aim to develop competence in school, sports, and other activities. Their ability to think on the level of concrete operations allows them to assess themselves and their environments logically. Also, they enjoy achievement, success, and peer recognition. Therefore, they want to experience success in their self-care efforts. It is in the school-age years that children become cognitively capable of taking responsibility for self-care. By the middle and late school years, the child should be able to make appropriate self-care decisions. It is a critical period during which the synthesis of cognitive skills and social responsibility can result in maximum self-care making decisions (p. 136).

By late adolescence or adulthood, persons have established systems of self-care. The self-care agency of adults is not constant. Changing demands lead to changes in self-care agency. Knowledge is required to choose which specific actions to take in a situation. When a self-care agent has no knowledge about a particular situation, that person does not know how best to act. Knowledge is developed over time particularly as an agent reflects on results achieved from prior action(s). Postexperience reflection is an intellectual process that influences future plans for deliberate action.

Though developed, the person must respond to changing therapeutic self-care demands through developmental stages of life, changing health-status, or changing conditions of living. In situations of altered health or illness, the self-care agency may be developed but not adequate for the therapeutic self-care demand, it may be in need of redevelopment, it may or may not be stabilized, or it may be declining. When the self-care agency is not adequate or operable, the person may need assistance in meeting the therapeutic self-care demand and/or in modifying the self-care agency. This can be in the form of dependent-care or nursing care.

An example of research that refines the first power components is Meyer's (2002) work on migraine headaches designed from the perspective of self-care agency. She developed a substantive theory of vigilance in women who had migraine headaches. The basic self-care requisite identified for women with migraine headaches was "the need to maintain function in the face of unpredictable bouts of severe headache pain and associated distress." One way women maximized their function was through the exercise of vigilance. Vigilance in women with migraine headaches can be conceptualized as the art of "watching out." Watching out, the core category in Meyer's theory has four subprocesses: assigning meaning to what it is, calculating the risk, staying ready, and monitoring the results. Watching out is a thought process that occurs as the woman scans her present condition for signs of an impending headache, a potential trigger, or indications that an existing headache is getting better or worse. The process of weighing the risk inherent in available alternatives is also part of vigilance, as is staying ready to intervene. The conditions related to the phenomenon of watching out are owning the label and making the connections. Watching out requires that a woman has identified herself as an individual who has migraines and has developed a set of connections against which to check her present condition. Strategies employed by the women as they watch out included learning from self and others. The consequences of watching out are choosing and implementing a course of action. Actions are chosen because the woman believes that they will optimize benefits over risks. Implementation of a course of action is done to maximize functioning.

INTENTION, MOTIVATION, AND CHOICE
AS PART OF SELF-CARE AGENCY

When the self-care agency is developed and adequate, the person must choose to perform the self-care actions, that is, to activate the self-care agency. The transitional operations of self-care agency include choice, intention, and motivation to act. All of these are instrumental or influential in the person actually taking the action chosen. A person can make a good choice, be motivated to act, and have the intention to act. But action will not occur until the person actually engages in the productive operations, takes the first step, and begins the process of evaluation or monitoring of the action outcomes to the intended. Actions are a function of motives and intentions that in turn reflect the personal beliefs and desires of agents.

A thoughtful plan for future deliberate action is called *intention*. It is an internal commitment to the choice made. Individuals often begin the day by thinking about what they intend to do that day—read a book, visit a friend, make an appointment. Beyond intention, moving this plan to action requires motivation and choice. One makes choices in determining the plan and in carrying it out. Intentions and choices require motivation to move toward action.

Motivation for action is well-studied in behavioral psychology and organizational behavior. An early model of motivation is Maslow's hierarchy of needs model wherein he proposes that if needs are not met at the lower level, there will be less motivation to act at the higher level. Another prominent theory is the self-determination theory with intrinsic (value-based rewards) and extrinsic (tangible rewards) motivators. The Web site *Changingminds.org* identified 25 different academic theories of motivation including attribution theory, cognitive dissonance theory, and goal-setting theory (*Motivation Theories*, 2010). The practical conclusion is that there are many different motivators for individuals, personal and social. To date there is no one model that best articulates with self-care deficit nursing theory. Orem proposed for additional study the consideration of the cycle of sensation and perception; appraisal, in terms of whether it's good or bad for me, and how this affects motivation (S. G. Taylor, personal interview, 1997).

In many social contexts, choices may express not preferences and the nature of the independent, bounded self but the nature of one's relationship with others. For example, one may make a choice for someone else. In this case, choice may signify one's care and concerns over the other person. One may also make a choice under close scrutiny by someone else and, therefore, feel constrained by social expectations. In these circumstances, the choice may signify one's need for approval from others—his or her concern over accountability. These and other interpersonal connotations can make the choice psychologically very different from the one made in the absence of any relational contexts and taken to be a 'pure' expression of ones preferences. (Markus & Kitayama, 2003)

On occasion, the person must weigh self-care values against other values and make a choice. Persons who choose to work in hazardous occupations, for example, in which they risk injury or disease, are giving less consideration to self-care than to certain job-related needs. These persons need to develop aspects of self-care agency to respond to increased demands for the universal self-care requisite prevention of hazards to life, functioning, and well-being. Self-care, while it contributes to life and health of individuals, need not be seen as the main purpose in daily life. While those of us in nursing and other health professions tend to view life through a health and/or self-care frame of reference, many others do not. In fact many persons view the world through economic, occupational, or family welfare perspectives first and foremost. What is viewed as important and of value forms the framework for thoughts and actions and gives meaning to experiences. It is this frame of reference that leads to the choices one makes. In some situations, the emotions of the immediate situation may affect the judgments made regarding action. This is often seen in end-of-life decision making.

It is also possible to deliberately choose actions that are not therapeutic and to ignore actions that are known to be helpful. Individuals at any given time may actively choose not to engage in self-care even when they have the functional ability to do so. Knowledge of the foundational capabilities and dispositions and power components of self-care agency helps us understand these choices to some extent, recognizing that the person has the right to make choices. They also have the responsibility to make good choices. Persons have action tendencies toward that which they appraise as good (liked). Three levels of good are described by Lonergan (1958, pp. 619–621). The first is the particular good, as opposed to bad. For example, it is good that I get a flu shot; it would be bad if I got the flu. A second level is the good of order, leading individuals to consider how their own actions are conditioned by existent arrangements, including patterns of relationships, and seeing their actions in relation to desires of others, as an aspect of human intersubjectivity. The third level is value or worth as the possible object of rational choices. Whatever is desired becomes a value when it is placed as a possible object of choice within a situation of action. This understanding of the levels of good "add another dimension toward respecting the practical intelligence of men, women, and children and their choices of what to do and what not to do before initiating concrete courses of action to change their life situations" in regard to self-care actions or any other action (Orem, 2001, p. 154).

SELF-CARE DEFICITS

A self-care deficit may occur as the result of changing therapeutic self-care demands and concomitant limitations in self-care agency. Or changes may occur in foundational capabilities and dispositions for self-care that limit the person's ability to respond to the therapeutic self-care demand. Self-care deficits are time and place specific. As therapeutic self-care demands change, the ability to respond to these changes will also vary. The person's awareness of some aspect of a self-care deficit, some self-care limitation, is the stimulus to act on his or her own behalf or to seeking assistance from another. This may be the result of on-going self-monitoring or the observations of another person. Sometimes the action response to the deficit may be as simple as seeking information, for example, I twisted my ankle, should I put hot or cold on it? In other situations a variety of experts or specialists could be consulted, for example, a nurse practitioner or physician for diagnosis and treatment of a health-related problem, a social worker when the limitation is related to resources or a family counselor when there are issues of relationships. Self-care limitations associated with self-care operations are factors or conditions that set limits on the person's ability for knowing, making judgments and decisions, and taking action. When these limitations are related to or articulated with a particularized requisite, it describes a self-care deficit or a component of a self-care deficit.

The therapeutic self-care demand defines the totality of action required and is derived from analysis of three sets of self-care requisites: universal, developmental, and health-deviation. The relationship of individuals' abilities to meet self-care and dependent-care demands can be more than, equal to, or less than what is needed. When the demand exceeds the abilities, a self-care deficit exists. When the abilities are equal to or greater than the demand, there is not an existent self-care deficit, though there may be a projected or potential deficit that can be identified.

$$TSCD > SCA = SCDeficit$$
$$TSCD \leq SCA \neq SCDeficit$$

A self-care deficit may be relatively permanent or it may be transitory. The self-care deficit may be overcome or eliminated, in part or wholly, if the person possesses the capabilities and can activate them. Otherwise, assistance from another may be necessary or desirable.

SELF-CARE LIMITATIONS

When self-care agency is not adequate to meet self-care requisites or when there are new self-care requisites, the person may experience self-care limitations, that is, things or situations that restrict the individual from providing self-care. Self-care limitations are elements of self-care deficit in that they express why the person is not meeting the therapeutic self-care demand. The limitation or inadequacy may be a result of a foundational capability or disposition or basic conditioning factor. A change in health-state typically brings about new self-care requisites. The limitation is usually seen in regard to the self-care operations and is known through an individual's self-appraisal of the self-care system, the environment, and self-management of that system of self-care within broader systems of living. Limitations are categorized in terms of restriction of self-care operations related to limitations of knowing, limitations of judgment and decision making, and limitations for engagement in result-seeking courses of action (Orem, 2001, pp. 279–282). Limitations of knowing may be due to absence or lack of required knowledge; limitations in knowing self and environment, and limitations in orientation and cognition for insights about the situation and for seeking to acquire knowledge. Limitations of judgment and decision making result because the person lacks an adequate knowledge base or chooses to avoid decision making situation's. Limitations for engaging in action may be due to the absence of some necessary condition for self-care and the conditions of living (Orem, 2001). The kind of assistance needed is defined by the identified limitation. Whether through a process of self-appraisal or an assessment done by a health care provider, the limitations that are identified direct the type(s) of action that will be needed. Exhibit 3.2 identifies the conditions and factors associated with limitations of self-care agency.

Knowledge, awareness, and understanding about the nature of the limitation and resulting inadequacy of self-care agency form the basis for the judgment that there is a self-care deficit, that there is a need for redevelopment or modification of self-care agency, or a need for

EXHIBIT 3.2
Conditions and Factors Associated With Limitations of Self-Care Agency

Limitations of knowing:
Set One
- Changed modes of functioning that are new and are not understood; lack of fit between what one has experienced and what one is experiencing
- New and unrecognized requirements for self-care associated with changed functional states
- New self-care requisites that are part of a prescribed regimen of health care that are not understood
- Lack of knowledge essential for performing the operations needed to meet specific self-care requisites, using specified methods and measures of care

Set Two
- Impairments of sensory functioning or perception and memory or attention deficits that interfere with the acquisition of empirical knowledge or recall of knowledge
- Disturbances of human integrated functioning that adversely affect empirical consciousness, cognitive functioning, and rationality associated, for example, with (1) organic conditions that are productive of toxic state, (2) mental and emotional illness, (3) brain disorders, and (4) effects of substances such as prescribed or unprescribed drugs

Set Three
- Dispositions and orientations that result in perceptions, meanings and appraisals of situations that are not in accord with reality
- Movement away from taking action to acquire new and essential knowledge
- Modes of cognitive functioning that affect mental operations associated with knowing when action is to be taken, adjusting action to existent or emerging conditions, and knowing when to stop action, and with organizing sets of actions into meaningful sequences toward result achievement

(Continued)

Limitations for making judgments and decisions:
Set One
- Lack of familiarity with a situation and lack of knowledge about appropriate questions for investigations
- Insufficient knowledge or lack of necessary skills for seeking and acquiring appropriate technical knowledge from individuals or reference materials
- Lack of sufficient and valid antecedent and empirical knowledge to reflect and reason within a self-care frame of reference

Set Two
- Interferences with the direction and maintenance of voluntary attention necessary to investigate situations from the perspective of self-care, for example, limitations of consciousness, intense emotional state, sudden or strong likes and dislikes, overriding interests and concerns
- Inability or limited ability to imagine alternative courses of actions that could be taken and the consequences of each

Set Three
- Reluctance or refusal of individuals to investigate situations of self-care as a basis for determining what can and should be done
- Reluctance to stop reflection and make a decision once a desirable and suitable course of action is identified and understood
- Refusal to make a decision about a possible course of self-care action or about the exercise or development of self-care agency

Limitations for engagement in result-achieving courses of action:
Set One
- Lack of knowledge or developed skills needed to operationalize decisions about self-care
- Lack of resources for self-care

Set Two
- Lack of sufficient energy for sustained action in the investigative and production phases of self-care
- Inability or limited ability to control body movements in the performance of required additions in either or both phases of self-care
- Inability or limited ability of individuals to attend to themselves as self-care agents and to exercise vigilance with respect to existent and changing internal and external conditions

Set Three
- Lack of interest in meeting self-care requisites
- Lack of desire to meet perceived needs for self-care
- Inadequate goal orientations and values placed on self-care that do not sustain engagement in the investigative and production actions essential for knowing and meeting therapeutic self-care demands

(*Continued*)

Set Four
- Family members' or others' deliberate interference with the performance of the sources of action necessary for individuals to know and meet their therapeutic self-care demands
- Patterns of personal or family living that restrict engagement in self-care operations
- Lack of social support systems needed to sustain individuals when self-care is complex, time-consuming, and stressful
- Crisis situations in the family or household that interfere with self-care
- Disaster situations that interfere with engagements in self-care and with the usual ways for meeting self-care requisites

Source: Adapted from Orem, D. E. (2001). *Nursing: Concepts of practice,* 6th ed., (pp. 279–282). St. Louis, MO: Mosby. Used with permission of Walene E. Shields, heir of Dorothea Orem.

assistance, and provide general guidance as to what actions to take. This may be the time when the person recognizes the need for professional assistance and seeks the help of the nurse. In a concern for childhood obesity, a mother might cut down on the amount of food served without making necessary adjustments in the nutrients provided. Without the child or other family members owning the need to modify the diet, they are likely to sabotage the mothers' attempts by eating snacks in other places. In conversation with the mother or one of the family members, someone might identify gaps in knowledge about the health-related situation, the misinformation or misinterpretation of information. In the present day of video sound bites or summaries of medical or research findings on the Internet, there is the potential for considerable confusion about the meaning of the findings and the application to the individual, hence the caveat to speak with the health-care professional that accompanies many of these reports.

INSTRUMENTS TO MEASURE SELF-CARE AGENCY

Measurement of self-care agency by the individual or another person is usually based on observation of behaviors, identifying insufficient or inappropriate actions or outcomes of action. The majority of instruments presented in the literature as measures of self-care agency are research tools and of limited use in clinical practice. These can be found along with the psychometrics of the instruments in

Connections: Nursing Research, Theory, and Practice (Young, Taylor, & Renpenning, 2001). They include the Self-as-Carer Inventory (SCI), the Assessment of Self-care Agency (ASA) and others available in the literature. Because of the complexity of the concept of self-care agency, it may be necessary to use more than one measurement instrument to get a complete representation of the concept in the population being studied. There are some measures related to developing self-care agency for persons with chronic illness where measurement is related to ability to care for self in altered health states. In many instances the measurement of self-care agency is related to the foundational capabilities and dispositions. Inferences from information about the foundational capabilities and dispositions are made regarding aspects of power components and/or self-care operations. If there is available information about the person's mobility, inferences can be made about the extent to which he or she might be able to manage the productive operations of self-care. Self-care operations are most directly measurable as they are the observable behaviors. Knowledge of a particular aspect of self-care can be tested by asking questions. Decision-making can be assessed by asking "if..., what would you do?" Manipulative skills can be measured by asking the person to do tasks. There is a need for development of clinical measures of *components of* self-care agency. There is a need, from a nursing perspective, to be able to measure components of self-care agency in relation to health-deviation self-care. Backscheider (1974) presented a model for measures of components of self-care agency related to a specific clinical population by identifying the tasks needed to manage diabetes and the aspects of foundational capabilities and dispositions and self-care operations associated with these. This remains a model process for clinicians and would serve well in the preparatory work for evidence-based practice.

A process for developing measures for identifying self-care and dependent-care requirements for children with asthma was developed by Cox and Taylor (2005). A template was created to perform four discrete but iterative cognitive and analytical stages; each stage reflected relevant self-care deficit nursing theory constructs. Stage 1 involved listing specific outcomes that could be expected when appropriate self-care/dependent-care actions had been taken. Stage 2 involved articulating all actions that a self-care/dependent-care agent would have to take to achieve each of these outcomes. In stage 3, each of the actions from stage 2 was categorized as either estimative self-care operations (thoughts), transitional self-care operations (judgments/decisions), or productive self-care operations (actions). In stage 4, questions were created that could be asked of dependent-care agents to assess competency with regard to each of the outcomes and actions (self-care operations). As a result of applying the template analysis process, four general action themes emerged that are now referred to as four ideal sets of action for pediatric asthma. Once the four ideal sets of actions were determined, each ideal action set was illustrated according to estimative, transitional, and productive self-care operations. This process is useful in developing models for evidence-based practice as well as tools for measuring aspects of self-care agency.

In many situations knowledge about the self-care agency and existing self-care system of a person is acquired through communication with the person or with family members. The nurse relies on a developed body of antecedent knowledge to evaluate and make judgments about the self-care capabilities of the individual.

Categories of self-care limitations can be useful in developing general models for describing interventions such as persons with limitation of knowledge acquisition. These limitations are less dependent on health-state and specific content to be learned but on such things as level of operative knowing. Section II describes ways of approaching some of these types of cases.

SUMMARY

The power and capabilities to perform self-care are identified in the science of self-care agency. When the requirements for self-care or the therapeutic self-care demand is identified, judgments can be made as to what the individual needs to be able to do to care for self. When limitations in self-care agency are present, actions need to be taken to overcome these limitations or seek assistance from others.

REFERENCES

Argyris, C., & Schön, D. A. (1974). *Theory in practice: Increasing professional effectiveness.* San Francisco: Jossey-Bass.

Backscheider, J. E. (1974). Self-care requirements, self-care capabilities, and nursing systems in the diabetic nurse management clinic. *American Journal of Public Health, 64*(12), 1138–1146.

Cox, K. R., & Taylor, S. G. (2005). Orem's self-care deficit nursing theory: Pediatric asthma as exemplar. *Nursing Science Quarterly, 18,* 249. doi: 10.1177/0894318405277528

Fan, L. (2008). Self-care behaviors of school-age children with heart disease. *Pediatric Nursing, 34*(2), 136.

Harré, R. (1998). *The singular self.* London: Sage Publications.

Inhelder, B., & Piaget, J. (1958). *The growth of logical thinking from childhood to adolescence.* New York: Basic Books.

Lonergan, B. J. F. (1958). *Insight: A study of human understanding.* New York: Philosophical Library.

Low, J. (1993). Perspectives on caregiving. *Canadian Woman Studies, 13*(4), 38–40.

Markus, H. R., & Kitayama, S. (2003). Models of agency: Social diversity in the construction of action. In V. Murphy-Berman & J. Berman (Eds.), *Cross-cultural differences in perspectives on the self (eBook): Current Theory and Research in Motivation* (Vol. 49). Lincoln, NE: University of Nebraska Press.

Meyer, G. A. (2002). The art of watching out: Vigilance in women who have migraine headaches. *Qualitative Health Research, 12*(9), 1220–1234. doi: 10.1177/1049732302238246

Moore, J. B., & Beckwitt, A. E. (2006). Self-care operations and nursing interventions for children with cancer and their parents. *Nursing Science Quarterly, 19,* 147. doi: 10.1177/0894318406286594

Motivation theories. (2010). Retrieved from http://changingminds.org/explanations/theories/a_motivation.htm

NDCG. (1979). *Concept formalization in nursing: Process and product* (2nd ed.). Boston: Little, Brown.

Orem, D. E. (2001). *Nursing: Concepts of practice* (6th ed.). St. Louis, MO: Mosby.

Wallace, W. A. (1996). *The modeling of nature: Philosophy of science and philosophy of nature in synthesis.* Washington, DC: The Catholic University of America Press.

Young, A., Taylor, S. G., & Renpenning, K. M. (2001). *Connections: Nursing research, theory, and practice.* St. Louis, MO: Mosby.

4

The Science of Human Assistance for Persons With Health-Associated Self-Care Deficits

*T*he third foundational nursing science is the *science of human assistance for persons with health-associated self-care deficits*. All persons experience a self-care deficit at different times and in different ways. A self-care deficit exists when the person's self-care agency is not sufficient to meet the on-going therapeutic self-care demand. The theory of self-care deficit is described as pertaining to persons with demands for engaging in self-care that they are unable to know or meet because of action limitations associated with their *health state* or *health care requirements*. The *theory of self-care deficit* is the essential element of self-care deficit nursing theory in that it is the presence of a health associated self-care deficit that establishes and gives direction to nursing.

The *theory of self-care deficits* includes the *science of human assistance for persons with health-associated self-care deficits. Health-deviation self-care* is action taken because of a specific health situation, such as illness or injury and thus not universally required of all persons, though at some time in life most if not all persons will experience health-associated self-care deficits. Furthermore, health-associated self-care deficits can include actual or potential limitations in knowing, judgment and decision making, and action in regard to health promotion, health protection, and illness prevention. Individuals in society, affected by human or environmental conditions associated with their states of health or their requirements for health care, may experience limitations in their ability to provide continuously for themselves the amount and quality of self-care they require. The theory of self-care deficit requires that the self-care deficit be identified and associated with a health state factor. Second, it recognizes that societies provide for persons who need assistance and includes an exploration of the kinds of human assistance needed when the person is not able to provide for their own self-care in whole or in part.

HEALTH

What is health? What factors can condition the self-care requisites to create a health-related self-care demand? What are the actions that need to be performed to meet those health-related demands and those universal and developmental requisites that need to be modified because of health factors?

There is no universally accepted definition of health. The World Health Organization (WHO) in 1948 (WHO, 1946) defined health as "a state of complete physical, mental, and social well-being and not merely the absence of disease or infirmity." Prior to this, health was commonly viewed as the absence of illness or injury. In 1986, the WHO modified their definition to include health promotion.

> Health promotion is the process of enabling people to increase control over, and to improve, their health. To reach a state of complete physical, mental and social well-being, an individual or group must be able to identify and to realize aspirations, to satisfy needs, and to change or cope with the environment. Health is, therefore, seen as a resource for everyday life, not the objective of living. Health is a positive concept emphasizing social and personal resources, as well as physical capacities. Therefore, health promotion is not just the responsibility of the health sector, but goes beyond healthy life-styles to well-being. The fundamental conditions and resources for health are: peace, shelter, education, food, income, a stable eco-system, sustainable resources, and social justice, and equity. (Ottawa Charter for Health Promotion)

The idea of complete well-being was interpreted by many as suggesting that we, as imperfect human beings, could never be in a state of health. Alternate models began to appear in the literature. Dunn's (1973) high-level wellness grid related health and environment to identify levels of wellness. A model for health promotion favored in the nursing literature is one developed by Pender (1996). Within Pender's health promotion model, health is defined as "the actualization of inherent and acquired human potential through goal-directed behavior, competent self-care, and satisfying relationships with others while adjustments are made as needed to maintain structural integrity and harmony with relevant environments" (Pender, 1996, p. 22). Another view or expression of the meaning of health is that it is

> a dynamic state of wellbeing characterized by a physical, mental and social potential, which satisfies the demands of a life commensurate with age, culture, and personal responsibility. If the potential is insufficient to satisfy these demands the state is disease. This term includes sickness, illness, ill health, and malady. The described potential is divided into a biologically given and a personally acquired partial potential. Their proportions vary throughout the life cycle. The proposed definition renders it empirically possible to diagnose persons as healthy or diseased and to apportion some of the responsibility for their state of health to individuals themselves. Treatment strategies [nursing interventions] should always consider three therapeutic routes: improvements of the biologically given and of the personally acquired partial potentials and adaptations of the demands of life. (Bircher, 2005, p. 335)

Health viewed from the person's perspective differs by basic conditioning factors such as age, developmental stage, and culture. The various aspects of health—physical, psychological, social—are inseparable in the individual. Although certain aspects of the person or the self may be isolated or emphasized for purposes of analysis or discussion, the person remains a unitary being and must be approached and treated as such. The individual's perception or subjective interpretation of his or her state of health must also be considered. This includes the person's acquired self-care agency, how they define their health states and their assigned cultural meaning of health state, and accept exhibit assistance.

Achieving and maintaining health is an ongoing process. Health from the perspective of early adolescents is seen as having six elements: absence of illness, physique, functional ability, health risk avoidance behavior, health promoting behavior, and holistic integration. Early adolescents' concept of health is a function of their cognitive development, moving from the more concrete absence of illness to the higher level of holistic integration. It is also a reflection of their family and cultural values and developing self-care system. How adolescents perceive health will condition their willingness to engage in healthy behaviors (Buck & Ryan-Wenger, 2003).

Elders' definitions of personal health can vary considerably and their perceptions of one's own health are not necessarily related to other measures of health status. A holistic and interlocking diagram of late-life health was constructed based on elders' statements. Table 4.1 depicts the three major categories showing that late-life health is multidimensional, and all elements are integrally linked to the perception of physical health domains and their characteristics emerging from elders' definitions of health (Damron-Rodriguez, Frank, Enriquez-Haass, & Reuben, 2005). Relevant models of health must allow for cultural definitions of quality of life and well-being and cultural influences on health. Similarly, meaningful concepts for middle-class majority Americans will not necessarily be relevant to other social groups; therefore, the models must allow for appropriate adaptation (Saylor, 2004).

TABLE 4.1
Emergent Constructs of Meaning of Health
for Ethnic Elders: Domains and Characteristics

CONSTRUCT	DOMAIN	CHARACTERISTICS
Physical	Somatic	Absence of illness Absence of symptoms Bodily functioning
	Physical Activity	Activities of daily living- walk, dance, etc.
Psychological		Positive attitude Gratitude Creativity
Spiritual		Religion Humanitarian beliefs Positive spirit
Social	Social Interaction	Family connectedness Support Interaction
	Leisure Activity	Hobby Music/art

There are many more detailed definitions of health in the literature, more than can be covered here. Two dominant themes, however, have meaning for self-care deficit nursing theory. The first is that evidence of holistic integrated functioning and evaluative judgments about health or not-health can be made by the self or others. Much of this evidence can be objectively measured; others can be identified by observation or self-report. Second, individuals have their own sense of health and well-being, their own definitions of health formed within a cultural context. What persons understand as health and what they value as to the functioning and integrity of the self affects the persons' self-care agency and conditions their self-care requisites as much as does the evidence of integrated functioning.

The acceptance of the definition by the WHO in 1948 had major impact on the direction taken by the health care system. This inclusive definition has led to significant differences in expectations of different constituencies regarding health care as a right or privilege. What should be covered by health care insurance? Definitions of health are significant in establishing professional boundaries and giving guidance to accept exhibit modes of intervention or interaction as well as for informing public policy debates including what is funded through local and federal initiatives.

THE CONCEPT OF HEALTH-ASSOCIATED SELF-CARE DEFICIT

The therapeutic self-care demand defines the totality of action required and is derived from analysis of three sets of self-care requisites: universal, developmental, and health-deviation. Universal and developmental self-care requisites need to be met at all times; failure to do so can have deleterious results.

Health state is a basic conditioning factor; it affects both universal self-care requisites and developmental self-care requisites and can also lead to an additional set of requisites, the health-deviation self-care requisites. As defined in Chapter 2, *health-deviation self-care requisites* are a unique set of requisites that arise from an altered health state and from methodologies used for therapy. Health-deviations may bring about feelings of illness or injury, a sense of discrepancy from normal. Management of health deviations or altered health states produce requisites that arise from the disease itself but also from interventions or medical measures prescribed or performed by health-care providers. Orem identified six categories of health

EXHIBIT 4.1
Health-Deviation Self-Care Requisites

1. Seeking and securing appropriate medical assistance in the event of exposure to specific physical or biologic agents or environmental conditions associated with human pathologic events and state, or when there is evidence of genetic, physiologic, psychologic conditions known to produce or be associated with human pathology

2. Being aware of and attending to the effect and results of pathologic conditions and states, including effect on development

3. Effectively carrying out medically prescribed diagnostic, therapeutic, and rehabilitative measures directed to preventing specific types of pathology, to the pathology itself, to the regulation of human integrated functioning, to the correction of deformities, or abnormalities, or to compensation for disabilities

4. Being aware of and attending to or regulating the discomforting or deleterious effects of medical care measures performed or prescribed by the physician, including effects on development

5. Modifying the self-concept (and self-image) in accepting oneself as being in a particular state of health and in need of specific forms of health care

6. Learning to live with the effects of pathologic conditions and state and the effect of medical diagnostic and treatment measures in a lifestyle that promotes continued personal development

Source: From D. E. Orem, *Nursing: Concepts of Practice*, 6th ed., p. 235 (St. Louis, MO: Mosby, 2001). Used with permission of Waylene E. Shields, heir of Dorothea E. Orem.

deviation self-care requisites. These are presented in Exhibit 4.1 (Orem, 2001, p. 235).

Orem uses the language of medical intervention and treatment in referring to diagnosis and treatment of altered health state. Medical does not refer only to physicians but includes nurse practitioners and other providers. When Orem was first developing her definition and concept of nursing, the 1948 WHO definition had just been proposed. The discipline of medicine was differentiated from other professions and disciplines by maintaining its proper object as persons with physical or mental disease and the diagnosis and treatment of the same. In the United States, with the broader definitions of health, the medical community broadened their scope of practice to include health promotion, preventive medicine, and some alternative therapies. They (M.D.'s) maintain their control over all these aspects of health care.

In recent years, there have been some hard-gained inroads into this domain by other providers—nurse practitioners, midwives, chiropractors to name a few; however, the language of "medical" remains. In the individual's quest to restore normalcy or reestablish the equilibrium, evidence of a health deviation leads to demands for determining what should be done. In the United States, this would generally be referred to as demand for medical diagnosis and treatment. From self-care theory perspective, seeking and participating in medical care for health-deviations are self-care actions.

The Diagnostic Process to Determine a Self-Care Deficit

When there is a need to determine the presence and nature of a self-care deficit, persons engage in a process of self-appraisal. This usually begins with an awareness of some limitation in their self-care practices, their health state, or their environment. They may or may not recognize this as a situation requiring self-care action. The initial concern is to identify the self-care requisite(s) being impacted by the situations. Joe finds himself unable to sleep through the night, waking up with a sense of not having rested. This sense of disequilibrium or discrepancy or deviation from normal initiates the diagnostic process for determining a self-care deficit. He is not maintaining a balance between rest and activity to restore, maintain, and promote activity foundational and essential to the life process. As he becomes aware of this discrepancy, he is exercising the power component of the "ability to maintain attention and exercise requisite vigilance with respect to self as self-care agent and internal and external conditions and factors significant for self-care" and initiating the estimative self-care operations. As he makes explicit the nature of the discrepancy or disequilibrium, depending on the level of developed self-care agency, he activates the self-care operations and attempts to take appropriate action. There are any number of events that can affect his diagnosis of the self-care deficit, including the antecedent knowledge and foundational capabilities and dispositions. Joe knows that being active and satisfied with social life is protective against insomnia at any age and promotes a sense of well-being and satisfaction with life in general. He also knows that drinking caffeine beverages in the evening have the potential to disrupt sleep. So Joe decides to go to the fitness center at noon and forego his after-dinner coffee. After a few days of doing this, he determines that this change did in fact improve his sleep and general sense of overall well-being. If his evaluation of the outcome of the self-initiated change in his self-care system did not resolve the disequilibrium, he might conclude that the actions he took were inappropriate or inadequate and reengage in the diagnostic process. Or he might conclude that his self-care agency is inadequate to meet the demand and seek professional help. The process of diagnosing the self-care deficit by the health-care professional is a similar process. It is described from the nursing or clinical perspective in Chapter 6.

HEALTH-DEVIATION SELF-CARE ACTIONS

What kinds of actions are required by a person experiencing an actual or perceived health deviation? What does one do when experiencing the need for specific forms of therapy such as medications or surgery? Are there common sets of self-care actions that can or should be taken? The NDCG proposed a general ideal set of self-care actions that persons will be required to take (NDCG, 1979, p. 283). These are presented in Exhibit 2.2. This structured general list is useful in identifying specific action protocols for persons with common health-deviations such as diabetes, asthma, hypertension, and so forth. In primary care and management of persons diagnosed with chronic disease, subset A is a critical element. It is difficult to engage persons in self-care and self-management if they do not "own" themselves as having an objectively established structural or functional state. Mrs. Jones is seen in the clinic by the nurse practitioner for routine check-up. The nurse checks her blood pressure and does other tests. She concludes that Mrs. Jones has hypertension and needs to take action to bring her blood pressure back to a safer level. In talking with Mrs. Jones, the nurse tells her that she needs to modify her diet and get more exercise. If that isn't effective, there may be a need for medication. Mrs. Jones's response is "I feel fine. No one in my family has ever had high blood pressure." As long as Mrs. Jones believes this, she will not participate in the recommended activities. Also, once she "owns" the health state, she also needs to "own a self" in need of a particular therapy. Only after that will she take the necessary actions, assuming that she has the knowledge and skills and motivation to perform and monitor the actions. Absent that, she will need assistance from someone with the necessary knowledge and skill to help her. Once a person has identified a health-deviation self-care requisite and initiated the seeking of assistance for the specific health problem, he or she will take responsibility for managing the technology to the extent possible within his or her self-care abilities.

SELF-MANAGEMENT OF HEALTH-DEVIATION SELF-CARE

Self-management is the process of developing, supporting, and directing the self-care system and integrating the self-care system into the over-all system of living. When a person has a chronic illness, "self-management includes the strategies that enable people to minimize their symptoms, share in decision-making about their treatment and gain a sense of control over their lives despite their chronic conditions" (Kendall & Rogers, 2007). Self-management is a process of "recognizing boundaries, managing the shift in identity and balancing demands." The purpose of these strategies is to create a sense of order in life, rather than the need to take responsibility for one's health. Self-management includes the mobilization of social resources and the maintenance of normal activities and relationships with family, friends, occupations and activities, despite their altered health status. Furthermore, individual strategies for managing health and illness cannot be separated from familial practices. Many family members view the tasks and activities associated with chronic conditions as part of family practice, rather than as the responsibility of the individual. In Australian indigenous communities, self-management has been redefined as collective self-management (Kendall et al., 2007). The social model of self-management respects the intricate nature of the ongoing lived experience and the security derived from family relationships in that they sustain a sense of continuity and a normal life (Gregory, 2005). This sense of normalcy and ontological security can also be found in collective peer support groups, particularly for those who do not have access to familial settings. Ontological security is a stable mental state derived from a sense of continuity in regard to the events in one's life; a sense of order and continuity in regard to an individual's experiences. People's ability to give meaning to their lives found in experiencing positive and stable emotions and by avoiding chaos and anxiety provide this security. Self-management enables people to not only direct their own lives, symptoms and treatment, but also to impact on the social context in which they live and the health services they receive (Kendall & Rogers, 2007).

There are several interpretations of the relationship between self-care and self-management. One is that the self-care system is a subset of self-management. This is valid when self-management is viewed in the broader context of daily living. Self-management within the theory of self-care is often referred to in the literature as *self-care self-management*. Other authors simply refer to self-management of some aspect(s) of an altered health state or modality of treatment. Sets B, C, and D of the ideal sets of actions propose the kinds of actions needed to reorganize the changing self-care system.

Research on self-management of medications has shifted from an early focus on adherence to the prescribed regimen and is now exploring ways to improve adherence or medication management. Simply adhering to a medication protocol is not necessarily good self-care. Persons need to know and be able to identify untoward side affects of a medication and take action if any appear. Possible actions might include calling the prescriber or the pharmacist, stopping the medication altogether or doing things to try to alleviate the symptoms. These actions may not be therapeutic, thus highlighting the need for working with the person to ascertain their self-care self-management capabilities. Successful self-management of medications has been shown to consist "of the following components: establishing habits, adjusting routines, tracking, simplifying, valuing medications, collaborating to manage, and managing costs" (Swanlund, Scherck, Metcalfe, & Jesek-Hale, 2008, p. 241). Two areas influenced the successful self-management of medications, namely living orderly and aging well. Besides management of medications, self-management of diabetes, arthritis, heart failure, renal disease, and other chronic diseases can be found in the literature. For diabetes, self-management is adherence to a self-treatment regimen that includes eating healthy, being active, monitoring blood glucose and taking medication, all critical factors in maintaining glycemic control. These can be affected by age, health status, diabetes knowledge, type of diabetes, duration of diabetes, self-care agency, and self-efficacy (Sousa, 2003; Sousa & Zauszniewski, 2005; Sousa et al., 2009).

Self-management is correctly viewed as a subset of self-care. Self-management is linked with an individual's ability, in conjunction with family, community and the appropriate health care professionals, to successfully manage the symptoms, treatment, physical, psychosocial, cultural, and spiritual consequences and inherent lifestyle changes required for living with a long-term chronic disease (Wilkinson & Whitehead, 2009). Ethically, nurses should practice with beneficence through provision of adequate training so a patient or individual can safely self-manage if they choose and have the capability to do so effectively. When there are limitations in the person's self-care agency, the nurse should not assume that the person can, will, or should take responsibility. Furthermore, research needs to be undertaken to fully understand the implications of expecting chronically ill individuals to undertake self-care management when health delivery systems, economic and social structures do not fully support this practice.

MODALITIES OF HUMAN ASSISTANCE FOR PERSONS WITH HEALTH-ASSOCIATED SELF-CARE DEFICITS

Helping

The type and degrees of dependence, the types of and individual variations in interdependence and interaction are often a result of the nature and duration of the health-deviation self-care requisites. In nursing, the assistance or help that is provided is also directly related to the health-deviation self-care requisites and factors conditioning the situation. The selection of methods of assisting is related to the situation and to the self-care agency of the person needing help. *Helping* another is an interpersonal activity. Though helping may occur between species (human-animal), in this context helping is referred to as human assistance. Needs for help are situation specific. Helping requires as a minimum two persons, one in need of assistance and another who can help. The helper needs to have knowledge of the person's need, the extent to which she or he can help, and what actions are practical in the given situation. Helping another is not always a simple process of seeing a need and responding. The helper may have the intention of doing good but not the knowledge and skill to accomplish that. Others have knowledge and skills and choose not to help. In the United States, there are "Good Samaritan" laws that protect helpers and those being helped. This legal principle is meant to prevent a rescuer who has voluntarily helped a victim in distress from being successfully sued for "wrongdoing." Its purpose is to keep people from being reluctant to help a stranger in need for fear of legal repercussions if they made some mistake in treatment.

Sometimes persons in need of help are reluctant to seek or accept assistance. They may not know what resources for assistance are available to them. They may minimize a need for assistance, thinking it's not serious or they aren't worth the trouble, "I don't want to be a bother." There are other factors that may influence the individual's acceptance of help such as cultural concerns or fear. When aware of these situations, the first action for the helper or potential helper may be to aid the person to recognize the need for help and assist them in finding the appropriate help.

Methods of Human Assistance or Helping Methods

The selection and use of one or more of the methods of assistance is accomplished in such a way as to ensure the validity of selection and use of the methods of assistance chosen by the helper. The method(s) selected need to be used appropriately so as to lead to the results sought. In most helping situations more than one of the methods of assistance is used, sometimes simultaneously.

There are at least five basic methods of helping. These are as follows:

1. Acting for or doing for another.
2. Guiding and directing.
3. Providing physical or psychological support.
4. Providing and maintaining an environment that supports personal development.
5. Teaching another (Orem, 2001, p. 56).

Each of the methods of helping requires interpersonal communication. The usefulness of the particular method of helping is determined by the result being sought. Good intentions aside, the helper must have appropriate knowledge and skills along with the ability to assess the situation before beginning to help. There is the potential to cause harm rather than good if the actions undertaken are poorly selected or applied inappropriately. Helping behaviors differ with regard to the degree of familiarity of the recipients and feelings of moral obligation to help. People are more apt to help someone they know and, in general, the closer the relationship the more likely that one person will help another, as within families. Helping behaviors can be viewed as a moral obligation; not only are individuals expected to look out for their own welfare, but they are expected to consider what is best for others. In western cultures, helping kin seems to be highly motivated by genuine feelings of obligation and is seen as a demanding but an obliging part of everyday life. In other cultures where a collective view is predominant, helping others is a natural part of life and a cultural expectation. When a person becomes a nurse, the moral obligation to help takes on special characteristics described as nursing ethics.

The identified helping methods are used in all human services. In different professions there is a greater or lesser emphasis on one or more of the methods. Often more than one method is used in the same situation. While acting for or doing for someone, the nurse can be providing psychological support and teaching. Traditionally, the hallmark of nursing care was acting for or doing for another, while at the same time providing support, teaching, guiding, and directing. With the expansion of roles and special areas of knowledge, this is changing. Much of the acting for and taking care of is now done by family or nonprofessionals, often under the direction of the professional nurse. Family members use the same methods when assisting one another. The selection and use of any of the methods of assisting can have physical or pschological effects on both the helper and person being helped. When a person is being cared for in the home, the resources for safety may not be available. The bed may be low, causing potential harm to the caregiver. There may be slippery floor surfaces that are hazardous. The caregiver may not have the strength and mobility needed to provide physical care. The person being helped may become dependent on the assistance and not develop self-care agency to the extent needed for the future. The distribution of care responsibilities between the person needing assistance and the one designated as helper requires consideration of three variables.

1. Individual requirements for care (demands), nature of methods to meet the requirements (tasks), and capabilities and limitations for providing that care for self.
2. The availability of a person or persons to assist in the provision of care and that person's capabilities and limitations in providing the care, including their own care requirements, and determination of their motivation and willingness to assist.
3. The environment within which the care will be provided.

Other factors that affect the selection of methods of assisting include the nature of the health deviation, the family system and relationships within the family, feelings regarding giving/receiving assistance, past experiences with helping, and so forth (Taylor & Robinson-Purdy, 1989).

Acting for or Doing for Another

When persons lacks the ability to take care of activities involving movement of the body, psychomotor skills, or more developed technical skills, they may need physical assistance from another person. The technologies used include assisting with all the various activities of daily living—bathing, toileting, moving from on place to another, eating, and so forth. Detailed descriptions of these methods can be found in fundamentals of nursing texts. Having a technically skilled care giver can be comforting, supporting, and therapeutic for the care recipient. Ideally, the person should be helped through all methods of assisting to assume more of their own care over time.

There are occasions when a person has the ability to care for him or herself but for therapeutic reasons should not and assistance is required to prevent hazards to well-being. Changes that are occurring in the U.S. health care system are placing a greater burden on persons and family members to take care of others at home. This is leading to a greater emphasis in nursing on the other methods of helping such as teaching, skill building, and support as ways to assure that the person will get the care needed. There is an increasing need for technicians to provide care to persons unable or limited in their ability to take care of themselves. The motivation for this is twofold: better outcomes for the person and reduced costs for the system.

Guiding and Directing

Persons who need to make choices may need guidance in examining options and selecting a course of action. *Guidance* by definition is assisting a person to "travel through," or reach a destination in an unfamiliar area, as by accompanying or giving directions to the person. This could refer to traveling through an illness episode or needing to make a decision about unknown or unfamiliar things. Further, the person may need or desire direction or supervision as they carry out the chosen action. Modalities for guiding and directing include using responsive language that gives reasons and explanations, validating feelings, modeling or demonstrating proper procedure, with direct explanation. Redirection of thinking, explaining logical consequences, negotiating and problem solving, active listening are also basic techniques for guiding and directing. *Directing* refers to more of a supervisory role, giving information or instructions for a course of procedure in an advisory capacity.

Support

Everyone who works with people gives supportive help at one time or another. Supportive help can be either active intervention by the helper in some crisis situation, or a kind of bolstering or palliative help to prevent further break-down in a chronic situation. This kind of support includes services to meet situational needs, protective services when indicated, moral support, and psychological support. The most commonly mentioned techniques described in the literature as supportive are

1. direct guidance and advice in practical matters;

2. environmental modification with the provision of specific and tangible services as needed;

3. provision of opportunity for the client or patient to discuss freely his/her troubling problems and feelings about them;

4. expression of understanding by the helper, along with assurance of interest in and concern for the patient or client;

5. encouragement and praise implying confidence in the patient's worth and abilities; and

6. protective action and exercise of professional authority when needed (Selby, 1956).

Psychology and counseling professionals differentiate supportive help from supportive therapy. Supportive therapy is aimed at supporting the strengths and constructive defenses of an individual in order that he or she may maintain a reasonably adequate social adjustment or achieve a better one. Effective supportive treatment results in the individual's greater comfort and freedom from anxiety and in his better social adjustment, which in turn may nurture his ego for growth. Supportive help has generally been thought of in terms of limited therapeutic goals sustaining an individual's strengths for reasonably adequate functioning rather than aiming for personality reorganization. From the perspective of nursing the selection of support as the primary helping method depends on the self-care limitations or deficits the person is experiencing, the environment within which care is being given, and the nurse's area of expertise.

Support also has a physical component. This idea of support comes close to the dictionary definition of the term "to hold up or in position; to bear the weight or stress of; to keep from sinking or falling; to sustain a load." This kind of support is an essential element in most acting for or doing for techniques. When a debilitated person is beginning to ambulate, the helper uses a safety belt to give support. Transferring a person from bed to chair is best accomplished if there is physical support.

Providing a Developmental Environment

An environment is considered developmental when it promotes or motivates the person to establish appropriate goals and adjust behavior to achieve results specified by the goals. It is the total environment that facilitates meeting the developmental self-care requisites. The nature of this environment varies with different stages of development. Physical conditions that contribute to development provide the necessities of daily life and for psychosocial and intellectual development. As a method of helping, support may focus on the acquisition of resources and ways of using available resources. The family and home are the primary developmental environments for the development of self-care agency and meeting of the self-care requisites. Parents structure environments to facilitate growth and development. Persons whose environments do not contribute positively to development may need support as well as assistance in making the environment conducive to development of the person and his or her self-care agency. Other methods of assistance may also be used to modify existing self-care agency and meet self-care requisites.

Florence Nightingale once noted that the art of nursing is to provide an environment in which patients are in the best position for nature to act upon them. Care settings with familiar and home-like physical environments can ease psychological stress and positively affect various health outcomes for patients. Environments providing space for relatives to spend time with patients, with exhibits and chairs for social interaction, have been shown to increase social contact between patients, relatives, and staff. The influence of health care environments on behavior and experiences has been studied mainly in environmental psychology. The physical environment of hospitals can convey different messages. The meanings of the environmental domain of nursing can include messages of caring and uncaring, stigma and social value. The environment can impose or ease suffering through experiences of cleanliness, location, space for interaction, and the presence of objects attracting attention. The physical environment influences experiences of providing and receiving care, and can be used as a nursing intervention. (Edvardsson, Sandman, & Rasmussen, 2006). Other aspects of environment that can be controlled and can have a positive affect are color, lighting, and sound. Long-term care facilities give particular challenge to the issue of a developmental environment. Limited visual acuity, hearing and mobility present problems for residents as does a constrained environment. The movement for "aging in place" is based on the importance of the environment for development in later life. Creating a developmental environment is accomplished not just with manipulation of the physical environment but also the effective use of the other methods of helping.

Teaching Another

Teaching another is a valid method of helping when persons need knowledge to overcome a self-care limitation or to develop a particular skill to be able to care for themselves. The desired outcome of teaching is learning, taking in of information so as to make a change in behavior possible and integrating the behaviors into the self-care system and the system of daily living. Teaching requires an understanding of the knowledge needs of the other, that is, the learner; including the present state of knowledge and the level of operative knowing of the learner. The teaching-learning process most in use is found in patient education programs established for particular health states or treatments. These are based on learning needs usually identified through a critical review of the empirical evidence. Evidence-based patient education programs need to be particularized or individualized; the more relevant patient education content is, the more likely it will be to produce changes in desired outcomes. Patient education is provided to guide the performance of self-care behaviors in the home environment. Patient education can take place in any environment. For persons with health-related self-care deficits, the health-deviation self-care requisites (Exhibit 2.1 in Chapter 2) and general ideal sets of action (Exhibit 2.2 in Chapter 2) provide a template for designing the content of patient education programs. The *content* for teaching another comes from the sciences of self-care, self-care agency, and self-care deficit. The *methods* used are from the learning sciences. After content knowledge has been identified, many teaching methods can be employed. More and more use is being made of digital technology and this will only grow, though for some this has its own set of challenges.

One way of creating learning that attends to broader development of capabilities is that of significant or transformative learning (Zubialde, Eubanks, & Fink, 2007). The critical dimensions of integration, humanistic development, caring, and self directed learning are essential for critical thinking, cooperative work, and problem solving in complex real life situations such as learning to manage a chronic illness. This type of "teaching" or educating is valuable when helping a

person develop or redevelop a complex self-care system. They identified six critical dimensions of significant learning:

1. Foundational knowledge that includes: (a) Appropriate conceptual
   and theoretical knowledge to understand a situation or problem
   (i.e., "sense making" knowledge) and (b) Accurate and practical
   information that guides action (i.e., "how to" knowledge).
2. Functional skills that provide the physical abilities, mental abilities, and tools that a person needs to successfully apply knowledge
   and effectively work on solving problems and attaining goals.
3. Integration skills that enhance a person's ability to: (a) See important
   relationships between knowledge domains and skill sets and their interdependence; and (b) Organize knowledge and skills to work across
   the multiple domains of complex problems (i.e., systems thinking).
4. Humanities skills that promote self awareness, social/cultural
   awareness, and enhance interpersonal relationships through:
   (a) Reflection on the rich personal, interpersonal, social, and cultural dimensions of life; (b) Experiencing and working with the
   personal and cultural models and belief systems that underlie our
   own and others actions; and (c) Building relationships that promote empathy, trust, and synergy.
5. Caring that promotes motivational and moral awareness and
   enhances one's ability to: (a) Appreciate and effectively work with our
   own and other's motivations, and moral/ethical frameworks; (b) Act
   in a sensitive manner to make a positive difference for self and others.
6. Self-directed learning skills that foster: (a) A desire to learn, grow,
   and adapt; (b) The ability to learn how to learn; and (c) The active
   transformation of beliefs, knowledge, and skills through a continual process of learning and growing (pp. 357–358).

Learning experiences that foster the building of capabilities in the
dimensions described above require a specific learning process that begins by using methods that help learners build an awareness of self, and
others, practical needs, and context through assessment, reflection, and
dialogue. Learners use that awareness to prospectively establish and
prioritize meaningful learning goals. Those goals then guide the learner
through the use of various learning activities to accomplish them. The
learning cycle then concludes with assessment and reflection on progress toward goals to further build awareness and launch another cycle.

CARE AND CARING DIMENSIONS FOR PERSONS
WITH HEALTH-ASSOCIATED SELF-CARE DEFICITS

Persons with health-associated self-care deficits may need assistance in meeting their requisites. The assistance provided is referred to as care. *Care* is the action that one person takes on behalf of another for the good of the other. The usual connotations of care relate to providing for, watching over, looking after someone. "I'll take care of you." "Take care when you drive in the rain." Care in the context of self-care deficit nursing theory refers to taking action to meet the requisites of the self or providing assistance to another to meet those requisites. When the self-care deficit is associated with health state, there may be need for nursing. The art and technology of nursing is found in the provision of care.

In Chapter 1, a nursing system is shown as having three dimensions one of which is interpersonal. The person-to-person relationships and interactions between nurse and patient constitute an essential element of a nursing system. These interactions occur within a societal frame. The societal aspects place individuals into varying positions and roles. The interactional aspects are dynamic; they are an instrumental means for the design and production of nursing care. They include contact, interaction, communication, and collaboration. The basic model for helping includes socioculture dimensions and interactional dimensions. The specific content of the help varies with the object of the profession. The interactional or interpersonal dimensions of helping situations are described by many as caring. Caring occurs when the relationship between the two persons is a "nurturing way of relating to a valued other toward whom one feels a personal sense of commitment and responsibility" (Swanson, 1993, p. 354) and applies to all caring relationships.

Caring is an important component in the delivery of nursing care. There are some nursing scholars and practitioners who claim that nursing is informed caring for the well-being of others, that the goal of nurse caring is to enhance the well-being of its recipients. The therapeutic practices of nurses are grounded in knowledge of nursing, related sciences, and the humanities, as well as personal insight and experiential understanding and knowing. It is the blend of knowledge/information and the goal of practice that distinguishes nursing from others whose practices include caring. In nursing, human interaction systems include reciprocal action and interdependence; wherein one knows the other as *you* and the self as *I*. Helping behaviors differ with regard to the degree of familiarity of the recipients and feelings of moral obligation to help. Five caring processes within the nurse caring relationships are described as:

1. maintaining belief in the capacity of others to make it through events and transitions and face a future with meaning;
2. knowing the range of responses humans have to actual and potential health problems in general and specific understanding of events as they have meaning in the life of the individual client;
3. being with, being emotionally present to the client;
4. doing for the other what they would do for themselves if it were at all possible; and
5. enabling the other to practice self-care (Swanson, 1993, p. 354).

In nursing, these five processes are informed by the intended outcome of client well-being. In self-care deficit nursing theory, the intended outcome is specifically expressed in relation to the self-care requisites of the client/person being helped within a legitimate nurse-patient relationship. In a meta-synthesis on caring, Finfgeld-Connett (2008) described caring as "a context-specific interpersonal process that is characterized by expert nursing practice, interpersonal sensitivity and intimate relationships . . . [the outcomes of which] include improved mental well-being among nurses and patients, and improvements in patients' physical well-being. . . . Nursing is perceived to involve an intimate relationship-centered partnership between the nurse and patient" (Finfgeld-Connett, 2008, p. 198).

Nursing consists of a unique relationship between patient and nurse, which is multifaceted and highly complex. Perspectives have ranged from caring as a human trait, a moral imperative, an affect, an interpersonal relationship (Finfgeld-Connett, 2007).

The relationship between two or more people (nurse, patient and/or family) is identified by Sumner as a moral ideal. Each person brings their historical and cultural background in a specific health/illness situation. The relationship will have cognitive, emotional, and attitudinal elements used to come to an agreement on an accepted course of action. The moral object of the relationship will be the patient's health. Both nurse and patient can acknowledge an "egalitarian ideal," though there is an inherent inequality in the relationship. The "temporary power of compassion" utilized by the nurse, along with the patient's own efforts regarding his/her health has the potential for growth and satisfaction for both (Sumner, 2001).

SUMMARY

Self-care limitations associated with health state may leave a person in need of assistance. General methods of helping were described in this chapter. The nursing practice sciences make these more specific and pertinent to nursing. Chapter 5 focuses on the meaning of relationships within the context of self-care. With the focus on self and person, one may lose sight of the fact that we become who we are in relationships and relationships sustain us when we are in need.

REFERENCES

Bircher, J. (2005). Scientific contribution. Towards a dynamic definition of health and disease. *Medicine, Health Care and Philosophy, 8,* 335–341.

Buck, J. S., & Ryan-Wenger, N. A. (2003). Early adolescents' definition of health: The development of a new taxonomy. *The Journal of Theory Construction and Testing, 7*(2), 250–255.

Damron-Rodriguez, J., Frank, J., Enriquez-Haass, V., & Reuben, D. (2005). Definitions of health among diverse groups of elders: Implications for health promotion. *Generations, 29*(2), 11–16. Retrieved August 2010, from Academic Search Elite database.

Dunn, H. L. (1973). *High level wellness.* Arlington, VA: Beatty.

Edvardsson, D., Sandman P. O., & Rasmussen B. (2006). Caring or uncaring: Meanings of being in an oncology environment. *Journal of Advanced Nursing, 55*(2), 188–197.

Finfgeld-Connett, D. (2007). Meta-synthesis of presence in nursing. *Journal of Advanced Nursing, 55*(6), 708.

Finfgeld-Connett, D. (2008). Meta-synthesis of caring in nursing. *Journal of Clinical Nursing, 17,* 196–204.

Gregory, S. (2005). Living with chronic illness in the family setting. *Sociology of Health and Illness, 27*(3), 372–392.

Kendall, E., Catalano, T., Kuipers, P., Posner, N., Buys, N., & Charker, J. (2007). Recovery following stroke: The role of self-management education. *Social Science Medicine, 64*(3), 735–746.

Kendall, E., & Rogers, A. (2007) Extinguishing the social?: State sponsored self-care policy and the chronic disease self-management programme. *Disability & Society, 22*(2), 129.

NDCG. (1979). *Concept formalization in nursing: Process and product.* Boston: Little, Brown.

Orem, D. E. (2001). *Nursing: Concepts of practice.* St. Louis, MO: Mosby.

Pender, N. J. (1996). *Health promotion in nursing practice* (3rd ed.). Stamford, CT: Appleton & Lange.

Saylor, C. (2004). The circle of health: A health definition model. *Journal of Holistic Nursing, 22*(2), 97.

Selby, L. (1956). Supportive treatment: The development of a concept and a helping method. *The Social Service Review, 30*(4), 400–414. Retrieved from The University of Chicago Press Stable URL: http://www.jstor.org/stable/30016000

Sousa, V. D. (2003). Testing a conceptual framework for diabetes self-care management (Doctoral dissertation. Case Western Reserve University, 2003), *Dissertation Abstract International, 64,* 3193.

Sousa, V. D., Hartman, S. W., Miller, E. H., & Carroll, M. A. (2009). New measures of diabetes self-care agency, diabetes self-efficacy, and diabetes self-management for insulin-treated individuals with type 2 diabetes. *Journal of Clinical Nursing, 18,* 1305–1312.

Sousa, V. D., & Zauszniewski J. A. (2005). Towards a theory of diabetes self-care management. *Journal of Theory Construction and Testing, 9*(2), 61–67.

Sumner, J. (2001). Caring in nursing: A different interpretation. *Journal of Advanced Nursing, 35*(6), 926–932.

Swanlund, S. L., Scherck, K. A., Metcalfe, S. A., & Jesek-Hale S. R. (2008). Keys to successful self-management of medications. *Nursing Science Quarterly, 21*(3), 238–246.

Swanson, K. (1993). Nursing as informed caring for the well-being of others. *IMAGE: Journal of Nursing Scholarship, 25,* 352–357.

Taylor, S., & Robinson-Purdy, V. (1989). *Assessing self-management and dependent care capabilities of hospitalized adults and caregivers in preparation for discharge.* Paper presented at the First International Self-Care Deficit Nursing Theory Conference, Kansas City, MO, October 1989.

Wilkinson, A., & Whitehead, L. (2009). Evolution of the concept of self-care and implications for nurses: A literature review. *International Journal of Nursing Studies, 46*(8), 1143–1145.

WHO. (1946). Preamble to the Constitution of the World Health Organization as adopted by the International Health Conference, New York, 19–22 June, 1946; signed on July 1946 by the representatives of 61 States (Official Records of the World Health Organization, no. 2, p. 100) and entered into force on 7 April 1948.

WHO. (1986). *The Ottawa Charter for Health Promotion. First International Conference on Health Promotion,* Ottawa, 21 November 1986. http://www.who.int/healthpromotion/conferences/previous/ottawa/en/

Zubialde, J. P., Eubanks, D., & Fink, L. D. (2007). Cultivating engaged patients: A lesson from adult learning. *Families, Systems, & Health, 25*(4), 355.

5

Theory of Self-Care in Relationships

No man is an island entire of itself;
every man is a piece of the continent, a part of the main; . . .
—John Donne

D emands for self-care exist within a person. When there is a focus on interpersonal units, the analysis of requisites and demands is modified. In the preceding chapters, reference is made to dependent care, to family, cultural groups, and community. Although humans are described as individuals, separate and unique, they live and survive by a series of interdependent relationships within the primary units of family, culture, and community. People come together for a variety of purposes and form groups. People who are not related as family may reside together for extended periods, such as in a partner relationship or a group home. There may be simple or complex relationships between individuals as in families or support groups as well as unrelated aggregations of individuals with no personal relationship, such as in an airport terminal or patients on a nursing unit. Relationships may be intimate and direct or impersonal. How health care or nursing systems are designed will take the nature of relationships into consideration.

The fundamental concepts of personalism (see Chapter 1) are participation, interpersonal community, and solidarity. Participation is at the foundation of personal existence. "There can be no individual, personal actualization without participation in the life of another . . . that is, in the life of another personal subject" (Donahue-White, 1997, p. 455). Participation also entails joining with others in shared activities, purposes, and goals and consists in engagement with others in the building-up and maintaining of community. The social philosophy of personalism can facilitate developing insight into the concept of multiperson units or situations.

Yang's (2003) conjoined model (Figure 2.3) places human needs within not only an individualistic perspective but also a collectivistic perspective where interpersonal needs take precedence in the genetic expression and genetic transmission needs. Yang identifies cultural differences in basic needs based on the interpersonal or collective. It is the collective that is of interest in this chapter. Yang suggests that not all human needs can be met by the individual, especially those related to genetic transmission.

UNDERSTANDING INTERPERSONAL UNITS OF CARE

Interpersonal units are comprised of two or more people. One of these is the dependent-care unit, which is an interpersonal unit but not of the same nature as other multiperson units. Orem considers the dependent-care system as an individual unit of care because the actions taken are directed toward the one who is socially dependent. Since the care system requires an interpersonal relationship, it is included here.

From the perspective of self-care deficit nursing theory, multiperson care systems are comprised of action systems serving the following purposes: (a) to meet the therapeutic self-care demands of members, (b) to facilitate the development and exercise of self-care agency of all members of the group, and (c) to establish and/or maintain the welfare of the unit. Existing individual care systems are viewed as subsystems of the multiperson care system (Taylor & Renpenning, 1995). These purposes are met through interpersonal interactions and self-care actions. The characteristics of human interaction systems as used by Orem include the overall conditioning effect of each person on the other person; the extensity, intensity, duration, and continuity of interactions; the differences in the aspiration of interacting persons; and the organization or lack of organization of the positions and roles of interacting parties (Sorokin 1957, pp. 436–452, as cited in Orem, 1995).

A unit is made up of more than a single person and regarded as a whole, as "we." The unit may range in size from two to some undetermined upper limit. In a multiperson unit, each individual has his or her own set of operations and requisites. Knowing the operations and requisites of each individual does not provide understanding of the functioning of the whole. Relationships between unit members to one another and to relevant persons outside the unit provide information about the functioning of the unit. The various action systems generated by persons in the unit must be identified and the various relationships need to be known if they are to have meaning for nursing or health care delivery (Taylor & Renpenning, 2001).

Human beings grow and develop in relation to other persons. "The Self exists only in dynamic relation to the Other . . . the Self is constituted by its relation to the Other; that it has its being in its relationship; and that this relationship is necessarily personal" (Macmurray, 1957, p. 17). The interdependence of human beings leads us to understand that the well-being or functionality of the unit can be an end in itself.

Humans have social instincts. They come into the world equipped with predispositions to learn how to cooperate, to discriminate the trustworthy from the treacherous, to commit themselves to be trustworthy, to earn good reputations, to exchange goods and information, and to divide labor. For most of us, our deepest sense of belonging is to our most intimate social networks, especially family and friends. As well as helping us to build a sense of self and individuality, such informal relationships also enable us to navigate our way around the demands and contingencies of everyday living. It is the nature of the relationships between people and the social networks of which they are a part that is often seen as one of the more significant aspects of community. In this chapter, three types of units are described and related to self-care deficit nursing theory: dyads, family, and community. A dependent-care unit has aspects of individual care systems and dyadic care systems.

THE THEORY OF DEPENDENT CARE

The foundation for dependent care is the inability of socially dependent individuals to provide their own required care. First introduced as a corollary to self-care, there is now a theory of dependent care presented for the purpose of further development and amplification. Knowledge of self-care is foundational to a theory of dependent care. Dependent-care theory is different from the theory of self-care in that it is the self-care deficit of the dependent that gives rise to the dependent-care demand and it is the dependent-care demand against which a judg-ment of the adequacy of the responsible person's dependent-care agency is made. The terms used in the theory of dependent care are distinct from self-care and are defined in Table 5.1.

The theory of dependent-care is complex. It parallels Orem's theory of self-care in a number of ways. Both self-care agency and

TABLE 5.1
Definition of Terms

TERM	DEFINITION
Dependency	A relationship between two persons in which one person requires something from another person. The legitimate basis for dependency varies as does the form or manifestation of that dependency within the social group.
Dependent-care agency	The complex acquired ability of mature or maturing persons to know and meet some or all of the self-care requisites of persons who have health-derived or health-associated limitations of self-care agency which places them in socially dependent relationships for care.
Dependent-care agent	"A maturing adolescent who accepts and fulfills the responsibility to know and meet the therapeutic self-care demand of relevant others who are socially dependent on them to regulate the development or exercise of the person's self-care agency" (Orem 1995, p. 457). The responsible person may be responsible by virtue of legal or social standing.
Dependent-care demand	The summation of care measures at a specific point in time or over a duration of time for meeting the dependent's therapeutic self-care demand when his or her self-care agency is not adequate or operational.
Dependent-care deficit	A statement of the relationship between the dependent-care demand and the powers and capabilities of the dependent-care agent to meet the dependent-care demand when that demand exceeds the dependent-care agency.
Dependent-care system	An action system produced in response to the dependent-care demand.
Dependent-care unit	A unit composed of the socially dependent person with limitations of self-care agency and the dependent-care agent or agents.
Social dependency	A condition that exists when persons require assistance from other members of society. It occurs with the context of a particular social unit. The provision of assistance and the nature of the assistance provided are a function of the general culture and culture of the specific groups.

dependent-care agency are capacities and capabilities for action, though the action or the intention of the actor is different in each instance. Limitations in ability to take care of self or dependent establish the basis for nurses to design and produce systems of care. Depending on the situation, a nursing system may be designed to address the self-care deficit of the dependent, the dependent-care demand, and/or the dependent-care agency of the responsible person. Like self-care, dependent care has its origins in people's requirements for regulatory care.

A set of premises about dependent-care was developed to place theory of dependent care in context (Taylor, Renpenning, Geden, Neuman, & Hart, 2001, p. 41).

1. Premises about persons in relation.
   a. Persons can only be satisfactorily defined in relationship to others and to the natural world.
   b. Human relationships are essential to physical and psychological development and ongoing relationships are essential for continuing development of the social self.
2. Premises about the interpersonal action system.
   a. The need for human interaction is ever-present and continuous. The nature of the interaction is dynamic.
   b. Actions systems between two or more persons have purpose and require exchange of information to achieve their purposes.
   c. In situations of family living there may be multiple subsystems of action including parenting and dependent care.
   d. The socialization of family members as self-care and dependent-care agents is a family function.
3. Premises about social dependency.
   a. Situations exist where dependency, which is where one person requires some form of assistance from another person, is expected and accepted by the social group.
   b. Dependent care exists within the context or frame of reference of social dependency.
   c. Throughout the life cycle the dependence may be related to age, development, and/or health state.
   d. There are degrees of relationship that can be identified as dependent, interdependent, and independent.

e. Conditions of social dependency may lead to a need for dependent-care systems.

f. Dependence may be instrumental (e.g., needing material assistance), emotional, or both.

The relationship between persons may be one of dependency. Social dependency exists when persons require or rely on assistance from other members of society. It occurs within the context of a particular social unit. The provision of assistance and the nature of the assistance provided are a function of the general culture and culture of the specific groups. Assistance may be provided by family, friends, or the larger community. Social dependency is distinguished from legal dependency, though in many situations the determination of legal dependence is an important issue. When one member of the unit is socially dependent on another, the relationship regarding care is more complex than the self-care system.

Dependent-Care Agency

The development of self-care agency and dependent-care agency is interdependent and occurs to some extent simultaneously within the context of ordinary living relationships. The development of self-care agency begins with the experience of being taken care of; I learn to care for myself, and at the same time I am learning to care for another. This parallel development is most obvious in cultures where dependent care is highly valued such as in the Mexican-American home where care of others is frequently demonstrated (Villarruel & Denyes, 1997). Some capacity for and engagement in self-care is necessary for dependent care.

Dependent-Care Unit and the Dependent-Care System

The dependent-care unit is made up of the socially dependent person with limitations of self-care agency and one or more persons acting as dependent-care agents. It may also include persons responsible for providing some aspects of care but who are not by definition dependent-care agents.

   The dependent-care system consists of courses and sequences of action that are being or have been performed by dependent-care agents in conjunction with the socially dependent person to meet the particularized self-care requisites of dependent persons. The dependent-care system is comprised of the interaction between the dependent and the responsible person. The dependent-care system is purposive, intentional, and influenced by the characteristics of dependency. The system has social, interpersonal, and technological dimensions. The specific actions that make up the dependent-care system are a function of the therapeutic self-care demand and self-care agency of the dependent; the therapeutic self-care demand, self-care agency, and dependent-care agency of the caregiver; and the interpersonal dimensions at the time of the provision of care.

In addition to the role of dependent-care agent, there is also the role of self-care agent to be performed. In designing dependent-care systems, these dual roles of the dependent care agent may be significant. In designing systems of care, both of these roles are taken into consideration. The articulations between these roles are shown in Figure 5.1 (Taylor & Renpenning in Orem, 2001, p. 285).

FIGURE 5.1   Dual Roles of Dependent-Care Agents

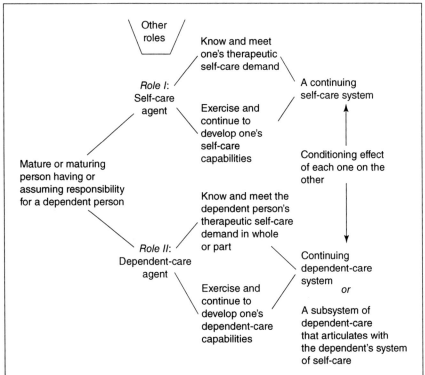

The Dependent-Care Demand

Dependent care is provided in response to a dependent-care demand through a system consisting of the actions of two or more persons, including the person in a state of social dependency unable to meet his or her own requirements for self-care and one or more responsible persons or dependent-care agents. In its simplest form, the dependent-care system consists of the actions of a dyadic unit where dependent care is a function of the therapeutic self-care demand and self-care agency of the dependent in conjunction with the dependent-care agency of the other (see Figure 5.2).

The following statements characterize the dependent-care demand:

1. Dependent-care demand is a function of the self-care limitations of the dependent.
2. Dependent-care demand is constructed from the self-care deficit; it is not the same in that it is a summation of care measures that require the actions of another person.

FIGURE 5.2   The Dependent-Care System

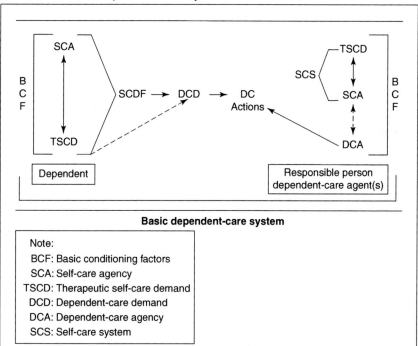

Basic dependent-care system

Note:
BCF: Basic conditioning factors
SCA: Self-care agency
TSCD: Therapeutic self-care demand
DCD: Dependent-care demand
DCA: Dependent-care agency
SCS: Self-care system

3. Dependent-care demand exists within the dependent and must be known by the dependent-care agent in order to develop a dependent-care system to meet that demand.

4. In situations where the dependent is mature or maturing, knowing the care demand is a joint action of the dependent and the dependent-care agent.

5. In infants and children, the expression of demand that is the basis of action is constructed by the dependent-care agent in terms of the particularized self-care requisites of the dependent.

6. In situations where the dependent is a mature or maturing person who is unable to participate in making known the dependent-care demand, the dependent-care agent constructs expression of the demand. This may require consultation from professionals.

7. Attributes of the dependent-care demand vary based on the nature of the relationship of individuals making up the dependent-care unit and the nature of the dependency, which may be related to age, developmental state, and/or health state.

8. The quantity and quality of dependent care required by an individual are a function of the complexity of the individual's self-care demand and nature of the self-care limitations.

When dependent care occurs within the family, it is a specialized family operation that requires management. The family is seen as the most common setting within which dependent care occurs and it conditions the dependent-care system (Taylor et al., 2001, p. 42).

The purposes of dependent care are meeting the therapeutic self-care demand of the dependent, through the period of dependency, promoting development, providing materials to sustain life, maintaining or developing positive relationships, supporting the individual, and in some instances, facilitating peaceful death. This is done through the dependent-care agent meeting the self-care requisites and/or regulating the exercise or development of self-care agency. If the dependent-care agent is responsible for managing care of requirements for more than one dependent, there is a need for that person to develop a system to manage requirements of all of the dependents. When the dependent-care demand exceeds the capability of the dependent and the dependent-care agent, a dependent-care deficit exists. The existence of a dependent-care deficit may be an indication of the need for nursing and is the criterion for nursing to become involved. The theory of dependent care articulates with the theories of self-care, self-care deficit, and nursing systems. In a dependent-care system, the dependent-care agent operates from a structured body of knowledge acquired through life experiences and information provided by various health-related professionals and other persons.

The Dependent-Care System

When the recipient of the care is socially dependent, a dependent-care system is established. Social dependency exists when persons require or rely on assistance from other members of society. It occurs within the context of a particular social unit. The provision of assistance and the nature of the assistance provided are a function of the general culture and culture of the specific groups. Assistance may be provided by family, friends, or the larger community. Social dependency is distinguished from legal dependency, though in many situations the determination of legal dependence is an important issue.

In addition to conditioning factors noted in the theory of self-care, basic conditioning factors in dependent care include the nature of the social unit, the relationship of the persons in the unit, the nature of allocation of roles and responsibilities in this and prior care systems, and the values of the family of origin. The quality and characteristics of the dependent-care system are conditioned by the capability of the dependent to communicate to the dependent-care agent information about sensation, perceptions, beliefs, and values. This information is made known when the dependent volunteers it. Other important information must be gleaned by the dependent-care agent's inquiring and observing. The quality of the communication conditions the nature and quality of the dependent-care system.

When more than one dependent-care agent is involved over time, the dependent-care system will be modified with each dependent-care giver, in part because of varying capabilities of the caregiver but also because of variations in the interpersonal dimensions of the dependent-care system.

There are specific tasks that the dependent-care agent performs. These are detailed in Table 5.2.

Taking a series of actions in an ordered way to meet the self-care requisites makes it a care system.

When the person is dependent because of age, such as a child, and that person also has an illness, there are a number of issues that arise regarding the development of self-care agency, dependent-care agency, and disease management. Child custody issues may involve

TABLE 5.2
Dependent-Care Tasks

CATEGORY OF TASKS	SPECIFIC TASKS
Tasks related to the other	Knowing and calculating TSCD of the other
	Contributing to developing the SCA of the other
	Regulating the exercise of SCA of the other (relates to operations)
	Responding to variations in exercise of SCA of the other
	Meeting the TSCD (or some component) of the other
	Systematizing the DC and SC actions into broader systems of living (e.g., family)
Tasks related to the situation of care	Determining the setting wherein care is to be provided
	Managing/modifying the environment
	Cooperating with other participants
Tasks related to the system of care	Maintaining the stability of the DC system including validation of the DC actions and system
	Communicating with other caregivers

both social and legal dependency concerns. An elderly person who is living alone may be socially dependent on a neighbor or friend for support and aid. In this situation legal dependence is not an issue.

The first consideration is the self-care demands and self-care agency of the child. The development of self-care agency is complicated by the need to integrate self-care related to an illness or injury with physical maturation and developmental events. The management of the illness and distribution of responsibility changes as the child becomes an adolescent, a period of life when control and independence are major development tasks. A major task for parents is determining how much responsibility should be turned over to adolescents or retained. These challenges can be particularly difficult for parents relative to their disease management responsibility because poor decisions can have life-threatening consequences. The complexity of decisions about who should be responsible for various aspects of disease management increases when there are two parents involved. The importance of the dependent-care performance of parents can influence the course of the illness and affect the future development of important self-care dispositions. Adolescents' failure to grow in self-care and deal with concurrent problems with illness control may be associated with parents' unwillingness to give up dependent-care responsibility or the premature relinquishing of dependent-care functions without corresponding assumption of self-care responsibility by the adolescents (Dashiff, 2003).

In designing dependent-care systems, the dual roles of the dependent care agent may be significant. In addition to the role of dependent-care agent, there is also the role of self-care agent to be performed. The articulations between these roles are shown in Figure 5.2 (Taylor & Renpenning, 2001, p. 285). In designing systems of care, both of these roles are taken into consideration.

MULTIPERSON UNITS OF SERVICE

Dyadic Units

The most basic of multiperson units is the dyad. There are two dyadic models that are relevant to self-care deficit nursing theory. The first is that of a care giver and a care recipient; the second is that of two people with a mutual shared relationship; the second is referred to as a collaborative or conjoined unit (Geden & Taylor, 1999).

The first model composed of a care giver and a care receiver depends on a mutually defined set of rules that govern their behavior (Coeling, Biordi, & Theis, 2003). This is descriptive of nurse-patient relationships in home care situations. A mutual dyadic entity could be one in which one party gives more than the other, or the care giver gives care for a reason different from that expected by the care recipient. In a mutually agreed-upon, dyadic care relationship a variety of conditions may apply over time, but the necessary conditions are that the dyadic parties agree, at any given time, to a mutually defined set of rules that govern their behavior. The rules of a caregiving/receiving dyad are those social constructions that govern the dyad's interactions as well as those of each of the people in the dyad such as found in the nurse practice act of a state.

The collaborative unit is a basic dyad that develops over time with care as only part or a facet of the on-going relationship. A collaborative care system exists within the unit; it is a purposive action system, a unique whole, with each member having demands and making contributions. It is greater than the two individuals' self-care systems or even the simple merging of their self-care systems. The collaborative care system is shared work resulting in negotiated roles for integrating and performing actions to meet the requirements for care.

The negotiation includes the identification of therapeutic self-care demands (individual and interactive) and the selection of actions based on individuals' capabilities for taking such action. Although the pattern or distribution of actions will vary in different units, the collaborative care system requires that both members make a contribution to the system of care. For instance, a couple may choose one member to be a primary decision maker about self-care and another may provide the material resources. This is unlike a dependent-care system wherein one person acts on behalf of another and there is no requirement that the dependent person actively negotiate his or her own care.

An interesting example of the development over time of a dyadic relational care system is that of the person with dementia and the partner/caregiver. At some future time, this could transition into the mutual dyadic entity. Dementia reinforces the interdependence of human life and highlights the fact that no one can flourish in isolation (Hellstrom, Nolan, & Lundh, 2005). Multidimensional and dynamic interrelationships between the person with dementia and his or her carer exist throughout the experience of dementia living. The person with dementia is best viewed as a social being. In most caring relationships the main motivation of the nonaffected spouse maintain the involvement of the person with dementia by creating ways in which their sense of agency and self could be sustained for as long as possible. Nolan, Lundh, and Hellstrom (2005) further highlighted the relational aspects of dementia and the work that is required to create what is termed a nurturative relational context in which couples (as opposed to individuals) actively manage the ways in which they live with dementia. In the case study they present, the couple clearly sees each other as having differing but complementary roles, which they actively discuss and agree upon. There is a growing realization that, in essence, "self" and "personhood" are often best conceived of as being created, constructed, and maintained within a relational context (Nolan et al., 2005). The most positive relationships are reciprocal and are based on an appropriate balance between independence, dependence, and interdependence. Valuing interdependence should be a central concern, that the couple could be the primary focus of the care system. Viewed from the perspective of a couple, a more nuanced understanding of the ways in which spouses do things together can emerge. They suggest a move beyond an individualistic conception of autonomy to one that is based on interconnectedness and partnership, recognizing the uniqueness of each individual while also acknowledging the interdependence that shapes our lives. This could lead to questioning the Western notion of autonomy as being the dominant value. As the person moves further along the trajectory of dementia, other persons may need to be involved in the day-to-day care of one or both members of the dyad.

The Family

A family is a system or unit of interacting persons related by marriage, birth, or other strong social bonds with commitment and attachment among unit members that includes future obligations and whose central purpose is to create, maintain, and promote the social, mental, physical, and emotional development of each of its members (Taylor & Renpenning, 1995). Family is a relational concept. Its existence is known through the unique and particular relationships among individual persons that meet the definition of family. There exists within the family a care system comprising many subsystems developed to meet the therapeutic self-care demands of the individual members through role allocation and interaction and some combination of independent and interdependent actions.

From the perspective of self-care deficit nursing theory, family has three meanings. First, the family is a basic conditioning factor, that is, a factor that influences an individual's self-care system. Self-care is learned within the family. The family conditions the specific values of self-care requisites. Maintaining a balance between solitude and social interaction can be a challenge in some families. Second, the family may be a resource available to be used by the individual for managing self-care requirements. It is the setting for infant and child care and for dependent-care systems associated with health-deviation care. Third, the family is a unit. The family has certain functions in meeting self-care and dependent care of all its members that are different from meeting each individual's self-care requisites. The family has the responsibility to prevent hazards and maintain normalcy as a unit, however that may look. The family has a unity, constituted from its members, that is substantially different in structure and function from the individual members. Family caregiving encompasses a wide array of cognitive, behavioral, and interpersonal processes and subprocesses (Schumacher, Beidler, Beeber, & Gambino, 2006). In some families, caregiving is the responsibility of one person; in others a network or roles and responsibilities develop.

Parenting

Parenting is a dynamic and learned process involving individuals, family units, and society. It is the rearing of a child or children by parent (father, mother, or person who stands in loco parentis). Dynamic, multifaceted, and complex, parenting is learned through role modeling by family, friends, and peers; formal classes; reading; and other informal means (Horowitz, 1994). Goals of parenting are to nurture, reassure, protect, comfort, stimulate, and promote the journey of the child from birth to adequate adult functioning or, legally, to age 21 (Horowitz, 1994). While there are relationships between parenting and dependent care, parenting is more than dependent care, and not all dependent care is done as a component of parenting.

Community

Community is a unit of identity; a name for an interactive group or aggregate of persons. A community can be understood both in terms of a geographical location (town, city, municipality, etc) or an interest such as church group or biking group, and a relational entity, which refers to qualities of human interaction and social ties that draw people together. It has been suggested that most people want to be part of a network of relationships that give expression to their needs for intimacy, usefulness, and belonging, and that people tend to self-segregate, that is, interact with others like them because of shared interests, similar cultural norms, and greater empathy toward individuals who remind them of themselves (Nilson, 1999).

Preserving the health of the community may be one reason people come together. There is a level of well-being that goes beyond that of the separate individuals to include the quality of interaction and the outcomes of those interactions on the unit as a whole. For the good of the family, members might have to do things they don't particularly want to do. There needs to be some agreement or understanding of the balance between the rights and responsibilities of the person and the others. Can a person refuse treatment for a communicable disease, such as tuberculosis, or refuse immunization against a dangerous disease such as measles or pertussis? Or does the group (community, society) have the right to require such treatment? Other interpersonal situations lead to similar conflicts, hence the need for laws and regulations, formal or informal, and cultural expectations.

Using metaphors developed by Kirkpatrick (1986), community can be thought of as an atomistic-contractarian model, an organic-functional model, or mutual-personal model. In the first, community is thought of as an aggregation, like a grouping of atoms, each driven by self-interest. The laws of the state (location) could require that you be immunized to protect your self-interest in not getting the disease. The second model describes community as a functional entity or system. Within this community there are continual interactions between the various elements of the system and subsystems with higher levels maintaining control of lower elements. Systems for distributing food for poor and homeless are an example. From the perspective of community, there would be concern about the availability of food, the quality of the food; if lacking, an appropriate action would be use of the political system to advocate for change. Finally, the mutual-personal model describes community as relationships. The location of the community or the common interests of members are secondary to relationships. Actions are taken not for self-interest or to maintain the functionality of the systems. It is taken out of realization that I cannot be what I am without another person. Persons have access to one another and are ready for one another.

From the perspective of self-care deficit nursing theory, community has several functions. First, community is a basic factor conditioning the self-care requisites of each and all the individuals within the referenced community, be it a community of place, interest, or mutual interaction. Using principles of public and community health nursing, community building may be a technology for designing programs aimed at the functions listed in Exhibit 5.1.

EXHIBIT 5.1
Functions of Community in Relation to Self-Care

1. Facilitating meeting the therapeutic self-care demand and dependent-care demand of community members.
2. Facilitating development and/or protection, and exercise of self-care agency.
3. Controlling environmental hazards and/or assisting community members to overcome the effects of such hazards.
4. Monitoring the health of members and preventing the spread of infectious diseases.

Source: From Taylor & Renpenning "The practice of nursing in multiperson situations." In Orem, D. E. (2001). *Nursing: Concepts of practice* 6th ed. St. Louis, MO: Mosby. Used with permission of Walene E. Shields, heir of Dorothea E. Orem.

SUMMARY

How we maintain our health and well-being extends beyond our own personal actions to those taken by us on behalf of others or by others on our own behalf. The patterns and means used are culturally determined or influenced. Future development of the self-care deficit nursing theory will benefit from development in the cultural and interpersonal areas. In the preceding five chapters, elements of self-care deficit nursing theory have been presented. Section II will translate these concepts into nursing practice.

REFERENCES

Coeling, H. V., Biordi, D. L., & Theis, S. L. (2003). Negotiating dyadic identity between caregivers and care receivers. *Journal of Nursing Scholarship, 35,* 21–25.

Dashiff, C. J. (2003). Self- and dependent-care responsibility of adolescents with IDDM and their parents. *Journal of Family Nursing, 9,* 166.

Donahue-White, P. (1997). Understanding equality and difference: A personalist proposal. *International Philosophical Quarterly, 37,* 441–456.

Geden, E., & Taylor, S. G. (1999). Theoretical and empirical description of adult couples' collaborative self-care systems. *Nursing Science Quarterly, 12,* 329–334.

Hellström, I., Nolan, M., & Lundh, U. (2005). "We do things together": A case study of "couplehood" in dementia. *Dementia, 4,* 7.

Horowitz, J. A. (1994). A conceptualization of parenting: Examining the single parent family. In S. M. H. Hanson, M. L. Heims, D. J. Julian, & M. B. Sussman (Eds.), *Single parent families: Diversity, myths and realities* (pp. 43–70). New York: Haworth.

Kirkpatrick, F. G. (1986). *Community: A trinity of models.* Washington, DC: Georgetown University Press.

Macmurray, J. (1957). *The self as agent.* New York: Harper & Brothers.

Nilson, G. E. (1999). Organizational culture change through action learning. *Advances in Developing Human Resources, 1,* 83.

Nolan, M., Lundh, U., & Hellström, I. (2005). We do things together: A case study of 'couplehood' in dementia. *Dementia, 4*(1), 7–22. doi:10.1177/1471301205049188

Orem, D. E. (1995). *Nursing: Concepts of practice* (5th ed.). St. Louis, MO: Mosby.

Orem, D. E. (2001). *Nursing: Concepts of practice* (6th ed.). St. Louis, MO: Mosby.

Schumacher, K. L., Beidler, S. M., Beeber, A. S., & Gambino, P. (2006). Transactional model of cancer family caregiving skill. *Advances in Nursing Science, 29*(3), 271–286.

Sorokin, P. A. (1957). *Social and cultural dynamics.* Boston: Extending Horizons Books.

Taylor, S. G., & Renpenning, K. M. (1995). The practice of nursing in multiperson situations, family and community. In D. Orem (Ed.), *Nursing: Concepts of practice* (5th ed., pp. 348–380). St. Louis, MO: C. V. Mosby.

Taylor, S. G., & Renpenning, K. M. (2001). The practice of nursing in multiperson situations, family, and community. In D. E. Orem (Ed.), *Nursing: Concepts of practice* (6th ed., pp. 348–380). St. Louis, MO: C. V. Mosby.

Taylor S. G., Renpenning, K. M., Geden, E. A., Neuman, B. M., & Hart. M. A. (2001). A theory of dependent-care: A corollary theory to Orem's theory of self-care. *Nursing Science Quarterly, 14,* 39.

Villarruel, A. M., & Denyes, M. J. (1997). International scholarship: Testing Orem's theory with Mexican Americans. *Image: Journal of Nursing Scholarship, 29,* 283–288.

Yang, Kuo-Shu. (2003). Beyond Maslow's culture-bound linear theory: A preliminary statement of the Double-Y model of basic human needs. In V. Murphy-Berman & J. J. Berman (Eds.), *Cross-cultural differences in perspectives on the self: Current theory and research in motivation* (Vol. 49, e-book). Lincoln, NE: University of Nebraska Press.

II

The Practice Sciences
of the Discipline of Nursing

Theories without practices, like man without routes, may be empty;
but practices without theories, like routes without maps, are blind.
—Gertzels, 1960

*I*n this section the nursing practice sciences, the link between nursing theory and practice, are explored. The nursing practice arena where practice knowledge is developed and validated is an untapped gold mine of information resources. However, as in the mining industry, finding that gold involves understanding the geology of the area and mapping it before being able to access the gold. So it is with the knowledge that nurses have developed over time, use every day, and that has become so important to daily practice. The nursing theories, foundational nursing sciences, and the nursing practice sciences provide guidance and a framework for structuring, exploring, and organizing information bits to become knowledge.

Nursing practice, theory development, and the reciprocal relationship between practice and theory has been a recurring theme in the nursing literature. The nurse is referred to by Ellis (1969) and others as *the practitioner as theorist*. At the time Ellis was writing, patient-care conferences to discuss situations of concern for which there were no ready answers regularly occurred in the clinical setting. "Nursing rounds" were held as teaching-learning opportunities. Nurses and sometimes other health care professionals presented their views, patients and family members presented their views, and small but significant advances were made in the development of nursing knowledge.

This knowledge was shared in the day-to-day conferences and rounds, a practice nursing would be well served in returning to.

In the ensuing years, the opportunities for nurses to pursue these learning opportunities in the clinical setting have gradually eroded. Less time, and in some cases no time, is included in the work plan and budget for patient-centered conferences, nursing rounds, and clinically focused continuing education opportunities. The role of scholar has been assigned to academia. This deprives nursing of the richness of the clinical environment as a source for developing and transmitting nursing knowledge. The importance of the practitioner as theorist, as developers of nursing knowledge, is reiterated in contemporary literature. A paradigm of practice-based knowledge production was proposed by Reed (2008), Reed and Lawrence (2008). This included promoting knowledge production in practice, promoting theoretical thinking, promoting use of clinical conceptual frameworks, promoting partnership for knowledge production, promoting attainment of baccalaureate and higher degrees, promoting the practitioner as clinical scholar. "The nature of nursing—involving daily encounters with the complexity, uniqueness, and the unpredictability of human beings' health needs—requires that nurses think theoretically and speak of their knowledge. Nurses look for patterns, make connections, posit possible explanations about their observations, test out and revise their ideas as the situation changes" (Reed & Lawrence, 2008, pp. 426–427).

The use of action research methodology applied to the study of the competing interests of the organizations providing care and of the professionals' concern for improvement of interpersonal care in long-term care institutions for elders is described by Dannefer, Stein, Siders, and Patterson (2008). Practitioners look for answers to the question "what can theory offer to individuals who are working simultaneously to transform institutional life while continuing to deliver services to the resident clientele on a daily basis?" (p. 104). In answer to this question, Dannefer et al. reported on the outcome of having nursing home residents, family, and staff forming Action Research Groups, which engage in exploring everyday institutional life, identifying practices and policies that can be changed. Elders, family, staff, and researchers together engage in action research but also are contributing to a reconceptualization of the concept of care incorporating "to be the one-caring AND the cared-for is a need of all human agents and actors." This example can easily be transferred to nursing, expanding our understanding of caring in the caring component of interpersonal relationships and other aspects of nursing practice.

In 1978 Carper published a seminal article "Fundamental Patterns of Knowing in Nursing" in which she described four patterns of knowing in nursing: (1) empirics, the science; (2) aesthetics, the art; (3) personal knowledge; (4) ethics. The socio-political was later added to these four (White, 1995). Knowledge development that will facilitate evidence-based practice requires exploring all five dimensions of "knowing nursing." Knowledge and theories related to the tasks that nurses perform are important but they primarily represent empirics. What of the other four dimensions? The groundwork for (a) pursuing a broad-based understanding of evidence for nursing purposes, (b) illustrating the links between self-care deficit nursing theory, the ways of knowing, and the contribution theories related to each of these ways of knowing could make to nursing practice, and (c) our understanding of evidence within a theory-based nursing practice frame of reference was laid by Fawcett (2002). Pursuing the reciprocal theory-practice process, it can be proposed that, by linking self-care deficit nursing theory and these five ways of knowing, there is direction for exploration of areas of practice which can expand knowledge, research, and theory development.

REFERENCES

Carper, B. A. (1978). Fundamental patterns of knowing. *Advances in Nursing Science, 1,* 13–23.

Ellis, R. (1969). Practitioner as theorist. *American Journal of Nursing, 69,* 1434–1438.

Fawcett, J. (2002, November 2–4). *Orem self-care deficit nursing theory: Actual and potential sources for evidence-based practice.* Keynote paper presented at the 7th International Self-Care Deficit Nursing Theory Conference, Atlanta, Georgia.

Reed, P. G. (2008). Practitioner as theorist. *Nursing Science Quarterly, 21*(4), 315–321.

Reed, P. G., & Lawrence, L. A. (2008). A paradigm for the production of practice-based knowledge. *Journal of Nursing Management, 16,* 422–432.

White, J. (1995). Patterns of knowing in nursing: Review, critique, and update. *Advances in Nursing Science, 17,* 73–86.

6

Nursing Practice Sciences

*T*he linkages between self-care deficit nursing theory and the ways of knowing do much to advance the development of nursing practice sciences. In Section I, the philosophical foundations of self-care deficit nursing theory and foundational nursing sciences were presented. The science of self-care with the theories of self-care, self-care agency, self-care deficits, and human assistance for persons with health-associated self-care limitations provide the basis for the development of the nursing practice sciences as shown in Chapter 1, Figure 1.4, The structure of the discipline. The nursing practice sciences are based in moderate realism where science is concerned with the study of real, where there is a distinction between knower and known using analytical and explanatory schemes and causal analysis and analogical reasoning (Banfield, 2002, unpublished). What research methods are capable of generating the knowledge necessary for the practical science of nursing within the self-care deficit nursing theory? Banfield proposed that empirical and interpretative methods may be appropriate. The researcher must have comprehensive understanding of the philosophy underlying the method, clearly identify the assumptions on which the study is based, justify the use of the method selected, and articulate how the study will contribute to the practical science of nursing. It goes with out saying that the researcher also needs a thorough understanding of the conceptual elements of the self-care deficit nursing theory. From the empiricist perspective, research methods or modes of inquiry include descriptive studies, case studies, descriptive correlational, and quasi-experimental as well as traditional experimental methods. From the interpretive perspective, ethnomethods, grounded theory, and phenomenological methods are also capable of generating knowledge.

The idea of a "science of the unique," focusing on the person instead of people, was proposed by Rolfe and Gardner (2005). Their proposals are made in a time when evidence-based practice in nursing is dominant. They argue that the traditional concept of evidence from formal research is merely the starting point for the on-the-spot generation of reflective/reflexive evidence by nurses themselves as part of everyday practice. The self-care deficit nursing theory is a science of the unique as well as the frame for all evidence gathering and interpreting the data, directing and facilitating its translating into practice as described in Chapter 9. Orem's theory provides a language for nursing. Every discipline has its own language elaborating the meaning of its phenomenon of concern, and the scholars of that discipline must know its unique language.

Nursing practice sciences have a twofold area of concern:

- *Intellectual knowledge* descriptive and explanatory of the nature, the structure and the results of nursing care systems designed and produced by nurses for persons seeking or under nursing care and
- *Nursing practice operations* necessary for the design, production, management, and control of systems of nursing care. These systems of nursing care may be for individuals or for populations.

DEVELOPMENT OF INTELLECTUAL KNOWLEDGE

Nursing takes place in an interdisciplinary environment. Shared health care goals are points of articulation between systems of care provided by nurses and by physicians and other health care personnel making up the interdisciplinary team of caregivers. However, within that interdisciplinary team, nurses have a specific contribution to make. Nursing seeks to answer the question *"How are the requirements for self-care and the production of the self-care systems of the individuals, members of dependent-care units, and multiperson units for whom care is being designed and delivered being affected?"* The purpose of the nursing practice sciences is to provide knowledge to answer that question. Practical science accepts the conclusions or results of other sciences as principles, using these principles to reach the ends of a specific practical science. Applying this to the nursing practical sciences, nursing would use principles from human physiology, human development, and other disciplines of knowledge to give direction to nursing, not just as a factual system which forms the basis for identifying more facts. For example, rather than accepting a list of basic human needs as facts, nursing would accept them as principles which leads to asking the question "to what use should these principles be put" for nursing purposes?

The world of the nurse is complex requiring a knowledge base drawn from anatomy, physiology, pathophysiology, pharmacology, nutrition, sociology, psychology, cultural anthropology, medicine to name a few areas. The questions become, where to begin, how to proceed, how to organize, and ultimately *what meaning do all of these theories and facts have for nursing situations and nursing practice?* The meaning that those theories and facts have for nursing becomes known as the relationships between conditioning factors and self-care requisites become known, as the relationships between therapeutic self-care demand and self-care agency become known, as the relationships between self-care deficits and nursing systems become known, and as comparable understandings are developed in relation to dependent-care and dependent-care systems. This knowledge development is the work of nursing practice sciences. This becomes the basis for evidence-based practice.

THE STAGES OF UNDERSTANDING NURSING

Self-care deficit nursing theory had its origin in practice as Orem sought an answer to the question "why does a person need a nurse?" Analysis of clinical practice situations has been central to the on-going development of self-care deficit nursing theory. In her writings and presentations, Orem has always stressed the importance of practice experiences in the reciprocal relationship of the development of nursing knowledge and the development of related theories. This relationship has been specified and made clear in the description of the stages of understanding nursing as shown in Figure 6.1.

FIGURE 6.1   Stages of Understanding Nursing

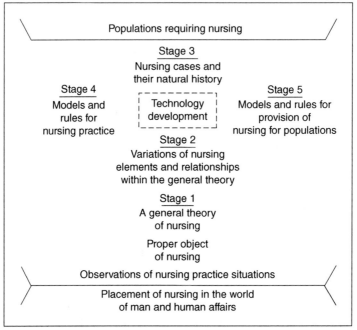

Source: Reprinted from D. E. Orem, *Nursing: Concepts of Practice*, 6th ed., p. 71 (St. Louis, MO: Mosby, 2001). Used with permission of Walene E. Shields, heir of Dorothea E. Orem.

Stage 1

The first stage in the development of nursing knowledge and related theories begins with developing an understanding of the human focus of nursing, the domain and boundaries of nursing, and beginning the descriptions of the subject matter of nursing. This occurs through observations of nursing practice situations, and consideration of the place of nursing in the world. This scholarly activity results in developing generalized understandings about the proper object of nursing, nursing as a human service, the place of nursing as a health service, and some sense of the subject matter of nursing. Stage 1 includes the development of a general theory of nursing such as self-care deficit nursing theory.

Stage 2

Stage 2 is the stage in which the conceptual elements of the general theory are validated and further developed. This includes specifying the nature and substantive structure of the elements, their relationships, and their articulation with facts and theories from fields of knowledge other than nursing. The substance of these two stages has been detailed in Chapters 1–5. In stages 3, 4, and 5, the nursing practice sciences are developed. Perhaps one of the most significant contributions of the second stage of development of understanding nursing and the contribution of self-care deficit nursing theory in particular has been the conceptualization and naming of the elements of concern in the theory, and the development of their substantive content. This has provided nursing with a language to describe the focus of its concern but more importantly it has provided nurses with a "short-hand" to talk about nursing. This becomes evident in analyzing practice situations when terms such as therapeutic self-care demand are referenced in analysis of a practice situation and the term reflects a consistent conceptualization of an area of concern to nursing embodying a human need, a goal to be achieved, and an action system to achieve that goal. More importantly these constructs can be incorporated into the patient record to reflect the concerns of nursing. The importance of this is underlined by Orem in the following quote "the lack of a nursing language has been a handicap in nurses' communication about nursing to the public as well as to persons with whom they work in the health field. There can be no nursing language until the features of humankind specific to nursing are conceptualized and their structure uncovered" (Orem, 1997, p. 29).

Stage 3

This is the stage of detailed investigation and description of nursing practice situations. The features characterizing each case, the patient variables in the situation, are identified and named. The factors that can condition the patient variables are identified and an understanding about the range of variation of the conditioning effects on the patient variables is begun. This lays the ground-work for development of models of nursing practice and development of classification of nursing cases.

Stage 4

Stage 4 is the stage of continuing development of models and general principles of nursing practice in relation to individuals, dependent-care units, multiperson units, families, persons in residences, and so on. These practice models and rules of practice provide direction for the diagnostic processes to determine the range of patient variables under specific conditions. Direction for specific nursing action and design models for systems of nursing may be included as part of nursing practice models—beginning to link practice and evidence.

Stage 5

Stage 5 is the stage of evidence-based practice. Nursing knowledge has progressed to the point where there can be identification and description of nursing cases by common features of patient variables that distinguish them from other nursing cases. Nursing can describe sub-groups or populations from the perspective of common features of concern to nursing. This "provides the basis for making inferences about appropriate nursing diagnostic, prescriptive, and treatment modalities; common features of nursing system designs, kinds of nursing results sought; and the values of nursing agency" (Orem, 2001, p. 172). The result is evidenced-based practice.

Developments leading up to and including stages 1 and 2 precede stages 3, 4, and 5. Stages 3, 4, and 5 may occur simultaneously. Also development in stages 3, 4, and 5 may lead to new understandings about stages 1 and 2. Theory development is dynamic not static—the input of practitioners is vital to maintaining this dynamic advancement. Specific examples relating to development of knowledge in each of the stages will be illustrated in the ensuing chapters.

TYPES OF NURSING CASES

Stage 3 of understanding addresses the advancement of nursing knowledge through the study and analysis of nursing cases. The categories used as organizers for analyzing nursing cases and describing areas of nursing knowledge have traditionally paralleled the interests of medicine—medical, surgical, psychiatric, obstetrical nursing. Disease entities such as cardiovascular nursing, rehabilitation nursing and areas of employment such as intensive care nursing, emergency nursing, acute care, long-term care, and community nursing have been and continue to be used as organizers in designing health care services including nursing.

Categorizing nursing situations using medical classifications has hampered the identification of nursing commonalities across medical diagnoses and clinical settings. For instance, although the medical specialties of cardiology and pulmonology are distinct from a medical point of view, there are many commonalities in the nursing require-ments for patients within these two diagnostic areas. Similarly, when setting is used as an organizer, the tendency is to think of nursing as community nursing, emergency room nursing, intensive care nursing, and so on, whereas there are many similarities in the nursing knowl-edge required to provide services in these settings. Separating provi-sion of nursing services into settings interferes with an integration of design and provision of service across agencies. Nurses did attempt to articulate some generalizations which crossed medical specialties and location of service through the development of "problem-based nursing." However, lack of a theoretical basis to provide direction in framing the problem limits the utility of this process for categorizing situations and cases from a nursing perspective.

The features of interest in nursing cases can be divided into two broad general categories. The first are the social, interpersonal, and technological features which focus on the persons of concern, who they are, their places in society, the roles each plays, the time and place of their interaction. The second are the characterizing features of the per-sons and their environments—the basic conditioning factors. Analysis of nursing cases involves identifying the characteristics of elements of concern with knowledge development occurring as recurring patterns within these broad categories are identified and cases can be catego-rized by commonly recurring features.

Early in their work the Nursing Development Conference Group (NDCG) began to work with the idea that the end product of nursing is a nursing system (NDCG, 1979). This led to the formalization of the theory of nursing system (Chapter 1). This theory provides direction for on-going analysis of nursing practice situations.

THE NURSING SYSTEM

The theory of nursing system is one of the most useful conceptualiza-tions for nursing practice. The theory of nursing system subsumes the theories of self-care deficit and self-care. (see Chapter 1, Figure 1.1). The nursing system includes the patient variables of self-care agency and therapeutic self-care demand and the nurse variable nursing agency. A nursing system has social, interpersonal, and technological dimen-sions. This has meaning for all of the ways of knowing as described by Carper (1978) and White (1995). The social dimension provides for recognition that both nurse and patient are members of a social environment with all of the ramifications that entails—family structure, cultural beliefs and practices, morals, ethical beliefs, socioeconomic environment, and so on. As an example of the impact of this dimension, and of new organizers being made available to nursing, the focus of nursing moves from *facts* related to social structure and to culture to the *actions and interactions* of nurse and patient in relation to social structure and culture.

Similarly, conceptualizing the nursing system as having an interpersonal dimension enables nursing to shift the focus from the patient as individual to the patient and nurse in action to achieve identified goals and to extend this to consideration of the interactions affecting health related self-care in multiperson situations. The new organizers become the goals to be achieved, the actions of nurses and patients/clients and the impact of these on the processes for meeting the therapeutic self-care demand and protecting/enhancing self-care agency. Verbal communication, touch, expressions of sympathy and empathy are among the ways the interpersonal system is operationalized. What meaning do these have for this patient? What meaning do these have for the specific nurse providing nursing? What are the implications for designing a nursing system when there are a number of nurses providing nursing? How do variations in differences in meanings between patient and nurse impact recovery of the patient when the patient's self-care agency is inoperable? These topics are explored further in Chapter 8.

The questions highlight the articulation between nursing and other disciplines of knowledge and are areas which require research and investigation from an interdisciplinary point of view and from the point of view of nursing as a discipline. Being able to answer these questions helps to move nursing from the invisible to the visible.

The technological dimension of the nursing system focuses on the action systems concerned with knowing and meeting the therapeutic self-care demand and relationships among the associated variables— self-care agency, therapeutic self-care demand, nursing agency. Through the processes associated with determining the relationship of therapeutic self-care demand to the self-care agency, the presence or absence of a self-care deficit is determined. The nature of the self-care deficit determines the type of nursing system required. There are three types of nursing systems. The nursing practice sciences correspond to the nursing systems and provide an "organizing framework for bringing together the essential features of nursing practice through which nurses generate systems of nursing care" (Orem, 2001, p. 175). Figure 6.2 illustrates these sciences and their elements.

FIGURE 6.2   Schematic Representation of Content Elements of Three
Practice Sciences

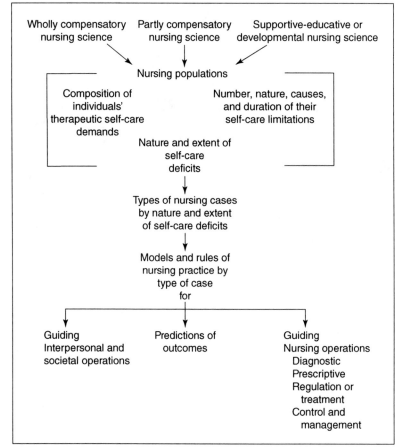

Source: Used with permission of International Orem Society.

NURSING PRACTICE OPERATIONS (NURSING PROCESS)

The broad parameters of the operations related to the professional-
technological components of nursing practice informed by all three
nursing practice sciences have the same foundation—human action,
the science of effective action, and the expressed proper object of nursing. All of these operations occur within a social and interpersonal
context. Specifying the aspects of the nursing system using the operations is referred to as design. Design is a core process of a profession.
Design is always a core component of operations. As a professional
intellectual activity, design requires both practical experience and

FIGURE 6.3   Elements of Design

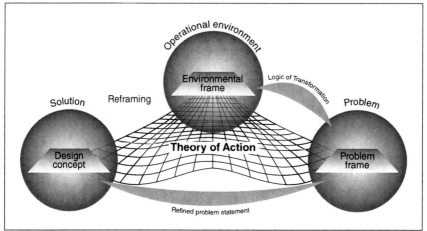

Source: Reprinted with permission from S. J. Banach and A. Ryan, "The Art of Design: Military Review," *Military Review, the Professional Journal of the US Army* (2009). Combined Arms Center, Fort Leavenworth, Kansas. It was originally published in the March-April 2009 issue of *Military Review.*

theoretical support. Banach and Ryan (2009) state that "mastery of a profession can only come through mentoring, coaching, and experiential learning as a member of a community of practice, in addition to the appropriate academic development of a leader throughout the course of a career" (p. 105). Design, planning and execution, and production are interdependent and continuous activities. Terms that have a specific meaning for the art of design include *problem situation, frame, reframing,* and *reflective thinking.* Design occurs in the context of situations, not problems. Designers determine their own purpose; therefore they set their own problems. Reframing shifts attention from trying to solve the current problem right to asking whether the right problem is being solved—naming is framing. The elements of design include understanding the operational environment, setting the problem, creating a theory of action, working the problem, developing a design concept, and assessment and reframing. Design applies to the individual practitioner as well as the organizations of health care (Figure 6.3).

It is important to point out that the conceptualization that nurses have about nursing is the force which guides their focus of concern. It provides the frame of reference for interpreting all aspects of the nursing situation. It influences which observations they make, the data they will collect, the meaning they will attach to the data, the course of action they will pursue in providing nursing care, the criteria for determining effectiveness of care provided, and the information they will add to their personal knowledge base. The meaning of this for nursing practice is illustrated in the following discussion.

The focus of the nursing practice operations is the relationship between the power of persons to perform self-care and the knowing and effective meeting of the therapeutic self-care demand. The nursing practice operations relate to the technological dimension of nursing practice and include diagnosis, prescription, regulatory or treatment operations, and control operations including evaluation. These operations occur within the context of the interpersonal relationships with patients/clients and within the contractual agreement. The operations are sequential but one may not be complete before another is begun. For example, the diagnostic process may not be complete before some regulatory action is begun. If a person is in acute pain and the cause of the pain is known, action may be taken to relieve that pain before proceeding further in the diagnostic process.

This conceptualization of nursing practice operations although embodying a problem solving process is not conceptually the same as the nursing process common in the nursing literature. The traditional understanding of nursing process has been as a problem solving process that begins with the presenting concern. This is followed by data collection related to that concern, branching out to other data indicated by the information gathered during the process of data collection, followed by selection from a list of nursing diagnoses which is most nearly consistent with the data collected. Continuing data collection and analysis is conducted to confirm or refute the selected diagnostic statement. Without a consistent theoretical perspective for framing the problem and providing direction for on-going data collection and analysis, there is limited opportunity for identifying organizers for development of knowledge specific to the discipline of nursing. Diagnosis and prescription have a different meaning when using self-care deficit nursing theory to frame practice as can be seen in the following discussion.

Diagnosis and Prescription

Nursing diagnosis is described in detail by Taylor (1991) and by Renpenning et al. (in press). From the perspective of self-care deficit theory, nursing diagnosis is seen as a process. This process is ongoing throughout the nurse-patient interaction. The result of the process may be a diagnostic statement or a diagnostic description. It forms the basis for prescription and regulatory action therefore addressing components of the therapeutic self-care demand, self-care agency, and the effects of conditioning factors on these variables. It involves a constant comparative analysis of the following relationships:

- basic conditioning factors, existent self-care requisite, and actions required to meet them
- effectiveness of persons' current self-care practices in meeting known components of the therapeutic self-care demand limitations that may interfere with knowing, decision making, production relating to self-care
- adequacy of power components to produce self-care to meet each component of the therapeutic self-care demand potential for future development and exercise of self-care agency.

The process of diagnosing the therapeutic self-care demand begins with answering the question:

Is there a need for immediate regulatory action? If yes, what action(s) is/are required?

For example, is there respiratory distress requiring immediate action. If there is a need, what action is required? Take action.

If the answer is no, then proceed to the next series of questions which are:

What conditioning factors are currently of concern?

For example: health state, therapeutic measures, family system factors, environmental factors, and so on.

Which requisites are currently being adversely affected by those conditioning factors?

For example, when there is a need for mechanical ventilation in addition to maintaining a sufficient intake of air, the following may need to be addressed:

- maintaining nutritional intake adequate to meet changes in metabolism associated with immobility and mechanical ventilation
- maintaining a balance between activity and rest
- contributing to prevention of ICU psychosis

In order of priority, what action(s) need to be taken to meet each self-care requisite being adversely affected?

Which requisites have the potential for being adversely affected in the future?

This is the first step in preventing adverse complications and one that is repeated many times during the care process.

When all known components of the therapeutic self-care demand have been specified, the next step is establishing the priority of the components of the demand and beginning the planning for meeting those components.

Diagnostic Processes and Self-Care Agency

The goal of the diagnostic process related to self-care agency is to determine the nature of the self-care limitations, the effect of self-care limitations that are present on the requirement for self-care capabilities and to evaluate the development, operability, and adequacy of *components* of self-care agency in relation to the therapeutic self-care demand. Note the use of the term components. Self-care agency is a theoretical construct. To be useful in practice, the substantial structure of self-care agency had to be understood. The initial work in uncovering the substantial structure was done by the Nursing Development Conference Group (NDCG, 1979). As described in Chapter 3, there are three categories of components associated with self-care agency. The diagnostic process associated with self-care agency involves all three areas.

The question to be answered: *is the person capable of meeting all of the components of the therapeutic self-care demand? If not:*

- Is self-care agency developed? Adequate? Operable?
- Are the self-care limitations related to one or more of the power components for self-care?
- Are the self-care limitations related to one or more foundational capabilities and dispositions?

From the perspective of self-care deficit nursing theory, "*all behavior has meaning.*" Compliance is not an issue.

Describing the Self-Care Deficit

The conceptualization of self-care deficit from the perspective of self-care deficit nursing theory is not the same as the term commonly referred to in nursing literature which refers to activities of daily living. A self-care deficit is said to exist when the value of the therapeutic self-care demand is greater than self-care agency. That is, the person lacks specific knowledge, is not making appropriate decisions, or is unable to perform the actions required in relation to health-related self-care.

The diagnostic statement(s) describe the relationship between the therapeutic self-care demand, and self-care agency, and may include information about the pertinent basic conditioning factors and/or self-care limitations. Unlike a medical diagnostic statement which is relatively stable, this statement is not static. It changes as the effects of conditioning factors on self-care requisites or self-care agency change or as self-care limitations change. It is important to note that from a moderate realism perspective, which is the philosophical basis of self-care deficit nursing theory, humans may guide change or take action by means of conscious purpose in light of rational experience. That action and thought are conditioned by circumstances but not determined by circumstances. In other words, the circumstances are not causal.

Some examples of statements describing the self-care deficit include the following:

- Extreme pain is interfering with ability to attend to learning needs.
- Anxiety regarding caring for self at home is interfering with ability to attend to learning.
- Permanent limitation of control of body and position limits ability to participate in self-care requiring movement unless and until substitute technologies are available, mastered, and employed.
- Learning new self-care measures will be affected by apparent inability to engage in concrete thinking.

Design and Planning

This phase of nursing activity incorporates what has traditionally been called "developing a nursing care plan" but examination of the elements of concern, the processes, and the product reveal that it is much more than that. The elements of concern are the current the conditioning factors in operation, the patient-related variables of self-care deficit, self-care agency, dependent-care agency if dependent care is involved; the nursing variable nurse agency; variables associated with other health care providers; the setting of the care situation. The product is the nursing system. The processes involve establishing:

- If there is action regarding any of the conditioning factors that can result in changing or eliminating the self-care deficit and if so how should that action be brought about.
- The regulation of self-care agency that is required and developing a plan for accomplishing this.
- Developing the action system and allocating roles to accomplish meeting the on-going components of the self-care demand.

If a dependent-care system is required, the plan should incorporate assessing dependent-care agency, identifying components of the dependent-care demand, developing a plan for protecting the self-care agency of the caregiver, enhancing dependent-care agency, and developing an action system to meet the dependent-care demand.

The use of the term *regulatory operations* provides direction for a different perspective on the role of nursing than is evident in the majority of the nursing literature. From the perspective of self-care deficit nursing theory and deliberate action theory, nursing is viewed as regulatory action and "nursing designs for regulatory care should (1) set forth relationships among the components of the therapeutic self-care demand that will result in good regulation of the health and developmental state of the patient, (2) specify the timing and the amount of nurse-patient contact and the reasons for it, and (3) identify the contributions of nurse, patient, and others to meeting the therapeutic self-care demand, to making adjustments in it, and to regulating the exercise or development of self-care agency" (Orem, 2001, p. 318).

This perspective recognizes that there are internally oriented self-care actions such as choice (choosing), which can only be performed by the self. There are also externally oriented self-care actions such as control of the environment. These may support internally oriented self-care actions such as those related to sleep, rest, and activity. A part of the system design may include measures to assist persons to limit or to engage in more self-care activity. The tasks to be accomplished in designing the nursing system include

- specifying the self-care tasks to be performed in a coordinated fashion within specified times
- making adjustments in constructing the ongoing therapeutic self-care demand
- regulating the exercise of self-care agency
- protecting powers of self-care agency
- providing for development of self-care agency.

Production of Regulatory Care

The production phase involves executing the roles that have been established in the design phase. This involves on-going interaction between all of the players—patient, nurse, and dependent-care agents—within and as they are influenced by the interpersonal and sociocultural frame of reference. The articulation of nursing systems with other systems of care becomes a consideration in the production phase. Systems of concern may be those related to other health care workers, to self-care systems, and to dependent-care systems. What is the relationship of one system to another? For example, in a critical care unit the medical system would most likely by the major system and the nursing system a subsystem. At the other extreme, in the home the self-care system or dependent-care system may be the major system in operation with the others being subsystems.

Control Operations

Control operations are concerned with establishing

a. if the plan as designed is being carried out
b. if the planned action system is still appropriate for the current conditions
c. "if regulation of patient's functioning is being achieved through performance of care measures to meet the patient's therapeutic self-care demand, if the exercise of patient's self-care agency is properly regulated, if developmental change is in process and is adequate, or if the patient is adjusting to declining powers to engage in self-care" (Orem, 2001, p. 324). This last quote from Orem has been included to show the breadth of concerns associated with self-care deficit nursing theory expressed only as Orem could.

The continuing development of the practice sciences is explored in the ensuing chapters. Compensatory nursing sciences which inform wholly compensatory and partly compensatory nursing systems are discussed in Chapter 8. In the wholly compensatory nursing system, the nurse role involves taking action to calculate and to meet all components of the patient's therapeutic self-care demand. If the patients are cognitively aware and able to communicate, they can participate in the judgment and decision-making components but the actual production of care is the responsibility of the nurse. The nurse acts for the patient to accomplish their required self-care. At the same time the nurse is responsible for supporting and protecting the patient not only in relation to meeting the therapeutic self-care demand, but also supporting and protecting developed components of self-care agency. Examples of such patient situations include caring for ventilator-dependent patients or for unconscious patients.

In the partly compensatory nursing system, actions to meet components of the therapeutic self-care demand are performed by both nurse and patient dependent on the patient's ability to participate. The nurse acts to compensate for the self-care limitations of the patient. The patient and nurse work together to regulate self-care agency. The patient accepts assistance of the nurse, and performs some actions as when a person is recovering from surgery or in the early stages of recovery from a myocardial infarction.

Supportive-developmental nursing science, discussed in Chapter 7, informs supportive-developmental nursing systems. In the supportive-developmental nursing system, the patients are capable of producing their own self-care but may need assistance with acquiring specific knowledge and skill or required guidance and support to accomplish meeting all components of the therapeutic self-care demand. The nurse and patient work together to develop and to regulate self-care agency. Note that the exercise of self-care agency is an internal operation which can only be carried out by the self. Regulation of self-care agency can be a joint activity of patient and nurse.

Understanding that the product of nursing is a nursing system has resulted in different conceptual and cognitive organizers being made available in the analysis of nursing practice, nursing cases, and the understanding of nursing situations. Doane and Varcoe (2005), working from a praxis perspective propose that theory development occurs every day in nursing practice as nurses try out, evaluate, and revise ways of thinking. This requires conceptualizing what is being thought about and naming those concepts. Working from an analysis of nursing practice situations, the originators of self-care deficit nursing theory identified and named the concepts that nurses were thinking about. The relationships among those concepts were proposed thus providing a structure to give some direction to theory development in practice.

All of the variables related to the three theories which are subsumed by the theory of nursing system and the variables associated with those theories and their interrelationships are now available for exploring nursing practice and for the development and structuring of nursing knowledge.

This forms the foundation for development of sciences of nursing practice. Identifying these variables in the patient record makes it possible to link elements of concern to nursing with other elements in the electronic record. This in turn makes possible the retrieval and analysis of information pertinent to nursing cases thereby turning bits of data into knowledge for nursing practice. The theory of nursing system and the continuing specification of its constructs and their relationships in reality settings provide the basis for developing models, rules of practice, and procedures for evaluating effectiveness of nursing systems—evidence-based nursing practice. On-going development of understanding of nursing systems rests in the development of the nursing practice sciences.

SUMMARY

This chapter has focussed on nursing practice with emphasis on the stages of understanding nursing by analysis of nursing cases and the development of nursing knowledge. An overview of the nursing practice operations in relation to the nursing system has been provided. In Chapters 7 and 8, these topics will be developed further in relation to specific types of nursing systems.

REFERENCES

Banach, S. J., & Ryan, A. (2009). The art of design: A design methodology. *Military Review, 89*(2), 105–111.

Banfield, B. (2002, November). *Research methods appropriate for development of knowledge related to the self-care deficit nursing theory.* Paper presented at the 7th International Self-Care Deficit Nursing Theory Congress, Atlanta, GA.

Carper, B. A. (1978). Fundamental patterns of knowing. *Advances in Nursing Science, 1,* 13–23.

Dannefer, D., Stein, P., Siders, R., & Patterson, R. S. (2008). Is that all there is? The concept of care and the dialectic of critique. *Journal of Aging Studies, 22,* 101–108.

Doane, G. H., & Varcoe, C. (2005). Toward compassionate action: Pragmatism and the inseparability of theory/practice. *Advances in Nursing Science, 28,* 81–90.

Grady, P. A. (2010). Translational research and nursing science. *Nursing Outlook, 58,* 164–166.

Nursing Development Conference Group. (1979). A general concept of nursing system. In D. E. Orem (Ed.), *Concept formalization: Process and product* (pp. 105–127). Boston: Little, Brown.

Orem, D. E. (1997). Views of human beings specific to nursing. *Nursing Science Quarterly, 10,* 26–31.

Orem, D. E. (2001). *Nursing: Concepts of practice* (6th ed.). St. Louis, MO: Mosby.

Renpenning, K., Bekel, G., Denyes, M., Geden, B., Orem, D., & Taylor, S. (2011, April). Explication and meaning of nursing diagnosis. *Nursing Science Quarterly.*

Rolfe, G., & Gardner, L. (2005). The science of the unique: Evidence, reflexivity and the study of persons. *Journal of Research in Nursing, 10,* 297–310.

Taylor, S. G. (1991). The structure of nursing diagnosis. *Nursing Science Quarterly, 4,* 24–32.

White, J. (1995). Patterns of knowing in nursing: Review, critique, and update. *Advances in Nursing Science, 17,* 73–86.

7

Supportive-Developmental Nursing Science

Supportive-developmental nursing science is rooted in nursing practice. It is concerned with the study of situations in which persons require assistance to identify, introduce, integrate, and manage new components in a self-care regimen for themselves or for a socially dependent person—the goal of nursing in primary care. The science is concerned with the relationship between the changes required, the capability to introduce those changes into the self-care system, and/or the nature of limitations interfering with the introduction of the change. Direction for exploration of these relationships is provided by self-care deficit nursing theory. Practice provides for further development of understanding of the relationships. The additional knowledge in turn leads to continuing theory development. This interaction between practice and theoretical development provides a structure for framing nursing practice in primary care and community settings.

The Institute of Medicine Committee on the Future of Primary Care defined it as follows: "the provision of integrated, accessible health care services by clinicians who are accountable for addressing a large majority of personal health care needs, developing a sustained partnership with patients, and practicing in the context of family and community." (Institute of Medicine Committee on the Future of Primary Care [IOM], 1996, p. 31). Geden, Taylor, and Ismaralai (2001) make this more useful for nursing by extending the definition to include "the outcome of the integration of sets of self-care acts into patients' systems of daily living" (p. 30). They go on to elaborate that *the unique contribution of nursing* to the interdisciplinary health care system is the focus on the patient's self-care system and assisting the patient with integration of self-care measures into that system.

The changes in self-care practices that are required may involve strategies to prevent adverse health-related conditions. They may be associated with controlling or regulating an existing health-related condition. There may be a need to protect developed components of self-care agency and/or to develop some new capabilities as a result of changes in the characteristics of one or more conditioning factors. Changes in foundational capabilities and dispositions and/or changes in the nature of the conditioning effect(s) on the components of the therapeutic self-care demand create the need for changes to the current self-care system. The changes required may range from minimal to extensive. In such situations there may be a requirement for a supportive-developmental nursing system. Very often when this type of nursing system is required there also is a dependent-care system in operation. In these cases the changes required in the self-care system may impact the dependent-care system as well.

Supportive-developmental nursing science is relevant to individual and multiperson units of service. It informs supportive- or developmental *nursing systems* when the individual is the unit of service. It informs the *nursing component* of supportive-developmental situations for multiperson units of service.

SELF-CARE LIMITATIONS

The role of nursing in supportive-developmental nursing situations is in relation to regulation of the exercise and development of self-care agency with the goal being to assist the person in integrating new self-care behaviors into the self-care system. The method of helping that is appropriate in each situation is directly related to the nature of the self-care limitation and the characteristics of the new self-care behaviors which are required. Types of self-care limitations may include the following:

- Changes in conditioning factors requiring adjustments in the self-care system. Examples include the onset of a chronic illness, changes in conditions of living, changes in economic resources, changes in family structure, and family system factors.
- A decline in self-care capabilities resulting in the need to learn new self-care strategies. Examples include deteriorating vision, decreased energy levels, change in physical capacities.
- The necessity of introducing a dependent-care system.
- Situations which require intervention at the community level such as services for physically disabled, crisis centers, adequate and safe food supplies, clean air, clean water, health care services, transportation, and so on.

THERAPEUTIC SELF-CARE DEMAND

The interrelationship of foundational capabilities and dispositions, conditioning factors, and self-care requisites results in the need to engage in certain self-care behaviors to accomplish health-related goals. When this interrelationship is stable, self-management takes place on a daily basis without particular attention being paid to it. However, when there is a change in the conditioning factors, there is a need to adjust the self-care system accordingly. One of the tasks to be accomplished in supportive-developmental nursing is to ensure that persons are able to calculate their own therapeutic self-care demand or that of the dependent person, to recognize when there is a need to adjust the action system required to meet that demand, and/or to recognize when assistance is required to accomplish these tasks.

Because the requirements for action (the self-care requisites) are influenced by the conditioning factors, all ways of knowing, *empirical, aesthetic, ethical, personal, socio-political* (Carper, 1978) are used by nursing in determining the therapeutic self-care demand. The importance of the meaning of knowing nursing in this way and integrating those ways of knowing into determining the characteristics of therapeutic self-care demand and associated requirements for self-care agency is illustrated in various ways throughout this book.

Exploring the range of variations in the therapeutic self-care demand in cases which are in the area of interest to supportive-developmental nursing science can lead to a classification system for these cases and ultimately to development of models and rules of practice for nursing. Can these cases be classified by age, for example, adolescents with *xyz* health state? Can they be classified by the requirement to modify the self-care system to integrate a particular therapeutic regime such as a medication management strategy? Foundational capabilities and dispositions such as vigilance or self-efficacy may be the basis for the categorization. It is possible that the organizer for classification could be a combination of the preceding suggestions as is required with the onset of a chronic illness.

Descriptions of patient tasks related to chronic illnesses and qualitative studies which describe the illness experiences from the perspective of the patient diagnosed with diabetes (Dashiff, McCaleb, & Cull, 2006), cystic fibrosis (Baker & Denyes, 2008), and heart failure (Artinian, Magnan, Sloan, & Lange, 2002) have been reported in the literature. Artininian et al. have conceptualized self-care behaviors within the perspective of self-care deficit nursing theory. In reviewing several of the other articles, it became apparent that although not named as such, some components of the therapeutic self-care demand were being described. Conceptualizing these as components of the therapeutic self-care demand provides for a broader understanding of the total situation. There is direction for exploring all of the self-care requisites to calculate the total therapeutic self-care demand thereby providing a more comprehensive view of the demand for action. There is direction for nursing to explore the characteristics of self-care agency that are required to meet the self-care demand and to develop appropriate nursing strategies. There is also direction for framing questions to be explored through formal nursing research programs thereby adding to the body of nursing knowledge. The utility of conceptualizing data from these articles as components of therapeutic self-care demand is illustrated in the section titled Types of Supportive-Developmental Nursing Cases.

EXAMPLE 1: Type I diabetes in adolescents

The developmental self-care requisite:

- *Integrate components of childhood diabetic self-care simultaneously with physical maturation and adolescent developmental events.*

Addressing developmental self-care requisites in adolescents requires that their interaction with universal self-care requisites be considered.

Changes in physical maturation associated with adolescence will affect the balance between caloric intake, exercise, and medication requirements. A changing palate and the influence of peer group tastes and habits will affect choices of food. Cognitive development, progression toward autonomy, parenting style, conflicts between teenager and authority figures, conflicts between adolescent and peer group are only a smattering of developmental issues which will impact determining what constitutes meeting this requisite. However, it does direct nursing beyond knowledge and skill development to consider where the adolescent is at developmentally and what their concerns and desires are, understanding their perception of the situation, looking for evidence of cognitive reasoning ability, exploring their value system, and understanding the influence of interpersonal relationships are all important in particularizing this requisite.

Consideration of this requisite also gives rise to questions related to self-care agency such as what indicators are there related to adolescent development that would indicate the adolescent could accomplish what is required? What kind of guidance and support is required under what circumstances? How can this best be provided? Should a peer group be incorporated into the strategies?

Evidence that nursing strategies are effective will go beyond assurance of adherence to prescribed protocols. The focus will move to the entire self-care system in operation.

Re Health Deviation Self-Care Requisites

The exemplar of concern is—manage insulin administration, adjust diet and exercise/activity level in relation to blood glucose level.

Questions related to associated components of self-care agency would include what are the characteristics of cognitive development that are required to enable meeting this requisite? What evidence is there of the following: adequate cognitive development, vigilance, ability to reason and make decisions within a self-care frame of reference? What other power components for self-care need to be developed in order for the adolescent to meet this component of the therapeutic self-care demand and what is the evidence that the state of development has been achieved?

The second exemplar of concern is—"deal" with emotions associated with having diabetes and being required to constantly manage the condition. Distress, anger, fear, frustration, depression, guilt have all been suggested as associated emotions.

Questions related to components of self-care agency include what coping skills does the person have? What coping skills need to be developed? How do persons acquire new coping skills? What

strategies can be employed by nursing to facilitate their development?
What behaviors will indicate strategies are effective?

EXAMPLE 2: Cystic fibrosis

In a recent study, Baker and Denyes (2008) studied predictors of self-
care in adolescents with cystic fibrosis. Their findings are significant
for practice in several ways, not only with adolescents with cystic
fibrosis but potentially for adolescents with other chronic health con-
ditions as well. They found the following:

- *Ego strength, sense of coherence, attention to health, health knowl-*
  edge, and decision-making capability all are predictors of self-care.
- *Attention to health and sense of coherence were predictors of self-care*
  associated with universal and health deviation self-care requisites.

These findings provide direction for nursing, specifically in answer-
ing the question, "what contribution can nursing make to support the
adolescent's attention to health and sense of coherence?" Strategies
suggested include engaging adolescents in conversations focusing
on their views of health and of what is happening in their bodies.
Encouraging family and friends to participate in these discussions
and make known to them the benefit of these discussions to the per-
son with cystic fibrosis. Programs can also be structured at a group
level or using the Internet for purposes of instruction or to develop
a support group. The efficacy of Internet support groups have not
been tested but the sheer numbers of young people who access them
when they are available is a testament to the potential benefit and
the influence of the peer group. Facilitating development of a sense
of coherence—a sense that life is meaningful and manageable—is
challenging. Active listening is a first step of communication. Helping
persons to become knowledgeable about required self-care and finding
ways to make that self-care manageable among competing demands
is a beginning step. This requires providing for on-going contact and
consultation. The findings could also be extended to consideration of
school nurses developing programs directed at teachers and students
to enhance development of ego strength, sense of coherence, attention
to health, and decision making throughout the school system.

EXAMPLE 3: Heart failure

The American Heart Association has published guidelines for promot-
ing self-care in persons with heart failure (Riegel et al., 2009). These
can be reconceptualized as components of the therapeutic self-care

demand. A sample of this reconceptualization and the implications for characterization of self-care agency is described.

Universal Self-Care Requisites

■ *Maintain current immunization.*

Do persons know what constitutes current immunization? Do they consider immunization safe, effective, and necessary? Are there costs associated with immunization that are prohibitive in the current circumstances? How available is immunization? What personal records are being maintained?

■ *Report presence of sleep disturbances to health care provider.*

What is the person's usual sleep pattern? Do they know the indicators of a disturbance that they should report to a provider?

Health Deviation Self-Care Requisites

■ *Incorporate taking of medications into daily routine.*

This involves initially obtaining the medication, planning for, and obtaining refills both of which require accesses to adequate resources including finances, contacting the pharmacy, and having some means of getting the medication from the pharmacy to the home. Is a visit to the health care provider necessary to obtain a refill? What is the person's understanding of the value of taking the medication? Do they know what changes are appropriate if side-effects occur? It also involves making appropriate adjustments to routine as a result of travel, illness, and conflicting obligations.

■ *Monitor for and manage incidence of edema. Weigh daily. Recognize significance of weight changes, report unintentional weight gain or weight loss in excess of three pounds.*
■ *Follow prescribed management instructions regarding dietary sodium intake and fluid restrictions.*
■ *Manage change to routines that may occur (travel, illness, fulfilling other obligations).*
■ *Follow prescribed diet—make adjustments to diet that occur as a result of unusual circumstances—for example, special celebrations, restaurant meals, illnesses.*
■ *Engage in regular exercise as prescribed based on individual characteristics.*

Meeting the above components of the therapeutic self-care demand requires that all power components of self-care agency be developed and operable. Some tools have been developed to assess development and operability of the components. More are needed. In addition, foundational capabilities and dispositions such as cognition may be affected when heart failure is present. There may be deficits in memory and attention. There may be alterations in executive function which result in faulty perception and interpretation of symptoms. These alterations in self-care agency may be a result of the pathology associated with heart failure, adverse effects of medication, or comorbidities. Is the person capable of recognizing these changes and taking appropriate action to compensate for them? The complexity of self-care in heart failure is well-recognized. In analyzing several studies conducted to try to determine what works in chronic care management for heart failure, researchers found that a multidisciplinary team composed of a variety of disciplinary providers engaged in face to face consultation when the patient's care provider was a participant was the most effective contribution to facilitating self-management (Sochalski et al., 2009).

Heart specialist nurses and protocols to direct their activities have been introduced into the health care system to address this specialized health concern. Concern was raised in one jurisdiction about whether protocol driven practice was compatible with the concept of patient-centered care. In a related study, researchers found that nurses' view of making their care patient-centered was accomplished by presenting to their patients that their heart condition was typical. They did not make inquiries about patient's priorities. The nurses' view was dominant. The researchers' suggested inquiry about the patient view should be incorporated into the nurse-patient interaction.

SELF-CARE DEFICITS

Self-care deficits in supportive-developmental nursing systems may be associated with lack of knowledge about actions required to meet the self-care demand of the current or projected future health care situation. Persons may have the skill to acquire the needed knowledge but lack access to the information or the means to acquire it. There may be cognitive deficits or emotional states which interfere with accessing or understanding available information. Cultural beliefs which are not consistent with the action system deemed to be therapeutic may interfere with appropriate knowledge being sought or appropriate action being taken.

There may be difficulty choosing from variety of options. The option chosen may be inadequate, inappropriate, or insufficient to meet the self-care demand. There may be misinterpretation of the actions required resulting in an inadequate self-care system. The person may lack sufficient energy and/or motivation to persist and in the required self-care actions over time for as long as required and/or to consistently perform the required actions. There may be difficulties associated with integrating new self-care activities into the ongoing self-care system.

Care in the first month after delivery of a first baby is a concern of nursing around the world. This situation provides a good exemplar for considering the concept of self-care deficit of interest to supportive-developmental nursing situations, particularly if breast-feeding is being implemented. The requisites of concern relate to universal, developmental, and health deviation self-requisites.

The following is a sample of what a new mother must attend to.

Maintain a sufficient intake of food and water to

- provide energy to care for self and newborn
- support postpartum healing
- facilitate establishment of an adequate supply of breast milk
- achieve appropriate body weight

Provide care associated with processes of elimination to

- reestablish normal elimination
- strengthen pelvic floor by integrating exercises into daily schedule

Maintain a balance between rest and activity and solitude and social interaction to

- have sufficient energy to care for self, child, and fulfill other responsibilities
- incorporate postpartum exercises into daily schedule
- Incorporate specific actions into daily routine to prevent infection of breasts, reproductive organs, and urinary tract.

Maintain family integrity and functioning

- Manage differences in relationship and role with partner
- Develop mothering role
- Integrate care system of new baby into family system

The question for determining the role of nursing becomes—*are the components of self-care agency developed, adequate, and operable in relation to the identified components of the therapeutic self-care demand.* Self-care deficits may be related to lack of knowledge, lack of resources, lack of skill, discrepancies between cultural belief systems and current scientific knowledge. They may be related to foundational capabilities and dispositions of vigilance, motivation, disposition to care for another and on and on. The wording of the above requisites has not incorporated cultural beliefs. This belief system may be a predominant factor in developing the action system.

Although each situation is unique, studying of cases and identifying commonalities in relation for example to existing or potential self-care deficits can lead to a basis for classifying nursing situations and developing models which can lead to rules of practice. For example, recognizing the widespread changes in therapeutic self-care demand and potential for self-care deficits can lead to community health organizations developing policies such as "mothers with first time newborns will receive a visit within the first 48 hours of discharge from community health nurses. The purpose of this visit will be to identify existing and potential self-care deficits and to develop an appropriate plan related action and follow-up."

TYPES OF SUPPORTIVE-DEVELOPMENTAL NURSING CASES

Supportive-developmental nursing cases are characterized by the following:

- The operational powers for self-management are developed and operable within stable or changing environments.
- There are limitations related to knowledge and/or skill development for meeting specific self-care requisites within an environmental context.
- A person is seeking to increase their competency in knowing and meeting their therapeutic self-care demand or to work with another in doing so (a dependent-care situation).

There may be variations by health state including specific disease entities, body system affected, expected length or duration, the extensity and/or intensity of conditioning effect and so on. The variations may also be by age and/or developmental state. Particular situations include onset or continuing concerns associated with a chronic illness. Developmental situations include changes in family structure—additions as in the birth of a child, or loses associated with the death of a family member, separation and divorce, children leaving home. The changes in developmental situations may be related to declining capabilities associated with normal aging or may involve extensive cognitive changes. In all of these situations, new self-care requisites arise with the requirement to develop new capabilities and/or coping skills. The nursing role reflected in the above cases is one that is expanding as care of persons moves from institutions into the community, as there is greater understanding of the relationship between self-care practices and healthful living, and as the role of the nurse within the health care system becomes more explicit.

Supportive-developmental nursing takes time. It is not something that can be accomplished by prescribing a drug or a rehabilitation exercise with a patient/client going home and following directions. It involves assisting the patient in making lifestyle changes, incorporating new ways of behaving into daily living. This takes a readiness to change. The following example is typical. The nurse practitioner had been working with a middle-aged overweight man with high blood pressure trying to help him to change his diet and increase his activity for several months. One day he came into the clinic and described an episode of tachycardia and shortness of breath which hadn't lasted long but which scared him. He said to the nurse "Now I get it." He was ready to work on new self-care practices.

DEPENDENT CARE

Very often in supportive-developmental nursing situations a dependent-care agent is also involved. The role of nursing in a dependent-care system is a function of the dependent-care deficit. It includes assisting in establishing the dependent-care system, helping the dependent person and the caregiver to recognize changes in the self-care deficit of the dependent, and facilitating development of new knowledge and skill in caring for a dependent because of changing effects of conditioning factors on the self-care requisites of the dependent or changes in their capabilities for action.

The dependent-care system is influenced by the extent of the development of the self-care agency of the dependent. In addition, there may be limiting factors particular to the caregiver. In addition to knowledge and skills related to self-care and to such care in relation to another, an egocentric orientation may interfere with a person's ability to see and understand a situation from another's point of view. There may be a reluctance or unwillingness to work with the body parts of another. There may be issues related to family functioning which interfere with production of dependent-care.

The theoretical basis for nursing in situations involving caring for a dependent family member is primarily addressed in literature associated with caregiving. This area is very complex because of the number of persons and variables involved. See Figure 5.2. The theory of dependent care (Taylor, Renpenning, Geden, Neuman, & Hart, 2001) provides direction for analyzing practice, providing direction in developing a conceptual framework for research endeavors, and organizing related nursing knowledge. Just having consistent names for describing the variables associated with dependent care facilitates developing a map to traverse this jungle.

In reading the literature associated with caregiving, there appear to be significant gaps concerning the caregiver, the recipient, and the interrelationships of the actions between the participants in the caregiving situation. The literature addresses caregiver burden, the processes related to caregiving, and the need for caregiver skill. However, as in nursing process when nursing theory is absent, the content and reasons for developing specific caregiving capabilities and executing specific caregiving actions is missing. Introducing the concept of dependent-care demand which is derived from analysis of the relationship between therapeutic self-care demand and self-care agency of the dependent helps to address these deficiencies. This content, the focus of the caregiving action, forms the basis for determining the dependent-care demand—"the summations of care measures at a specific point in time or over a duration of time for meeting the dependent's therapeutic self-care demand when his or her self-care agency is not adequate or operational" (Taylor et al., 2001, p. 40). This provides the basis for identification of the knowledge and skill required for caregiving situations, direction for understanding the context in which the care is provided, and the impact of that context on the skills and processes involved.

In studies related to family caregivers of persons with cancer, Schumacher, Stewart, Archbold, Dodd, and Dibble (2000) describe the development of the concept family caregiving skill, identifying that some caregivers "do" caregiving better than others and address the need for nurses to identify what factors make the difference. These authors go on to address the need to understand this process better so that tools can be developed which would assist nurses to asses caregiving skills.

In a subsequent article the construct of caregiving skill was reconceptualized as caregiver skill (Schumacher, Beidler, Beeber, & Gambino, 2006). This reconceptualization changed the focus of attention from the person providing the care to the processes associated with the care. However, as "theories without practices, like man without routes, may be empty; but practices without theories, like routes without maps, are blind" so processes require theories. Ultimately, in the process of data analysis, the researchers defined family caregiving as a "process that occurs in response to an illness and encompasses multiple cognitive, behavioral, and interpersonal processes." Caregiving skill was defined as "the ability to respond effectively and smoothly to the demands of the illness and pattern of care using these processes." This incorporation of demands of the illness situation and the interaction between the demands arising from the illness and the requirement for care is consistent with the basic understandings associated with the theory of dependent care—specifically the construct of dependent-care demand and understanding that caregiving occurs within an interpersonal frame of reference which influences not only the actions required but the results of those actions. However, the missing piece, still to be formalized by nursing science, is the detail related to the totality of the therapeutic self-care demand of persons receiving treatment for cancer, the self-care deficit, the dependent-care deficit, and ultimately the assessment of family "caregiving skills."

In the meantime, self-care deficit nursing theory provides direction for development of discharge instructions for persons with cancer and for their caregivers. The caregiving processes that have been identified in the literature include monitoring, interpreting, making decisions, taking action, making adjustments. The content associated with those processes can be determined by linking the conditioning effects of the cancer treatment with the self-care requisites affected by the specific treatment. In general, treatment for cancer impacts the following requisites:

- Maintaining a sufficient intake of food and water
- Maintaining a balance between rest and activity and solitude and social interaction
- Prevention of hazards
- Promotion of normalcy
- Overcoming factors which interfere with development

■ Securing medical assistance
■ Being aware of and attending to pathologic conditions and states
■ Carrying out diagnostic, therapeutic, and rehabilitation measures
■ Attending to comfort
■ Modifying self-concept
■ Modifying lifestyle

Specifying the content for these processes involves the following:

■ Determining the conditioning effect of various treatments for specific forms of cancer on specific self-care requisites
■ Developing specific goals to be achieved for these requisites, for
example, maintaining a sufficient intake of food, monitoring for de-
terioration in condition, reporting significant changes to appropriate person
■ (Specify how this will be achieved) Providing a diet with specific
caloric intake of required consistency, monitor daily intake, and keep
a record of days when person does not eat, check weight weekly,
report to physician/nurse if weight loss has exceeded three pounds
■ Evaluating caregivers' capability in reference to the specifications of
the actions required—do they understand importance of monitoring weight, are they likely to do this, does the family have a scale,
do they know who to contact regarding changes

The difference that self-care deficit nursing theory makes in the above
situation is the direction for identifying content to achieve the required self-care/dependent care—what is required, the action system
to achieve what is required, evaluating capability for producing the
required actions. There is also direction for evaluating the extent to
which the goals are being achieved and the effectiveness of nursing
involvement.

BEYOND THE INDIVIDUAL—MULTIPERSON UNITS OF SERVICE

Self-care deficit nursing theory also provides direction for nursing in
situations

■ where the individual has responsibility to influence the environmental context
■ in situations where it is the responsibility of a social group to influence the environmental context

■ in situations where it is the responsibility of society at large to manage environmental context through one or more of public policy, education, legislation, provision of required resources

In these situations, it may be that a multiperson unit is the service unit of concern to nursing. In such situations, the *system* of care is no longer a nursing system but an interdisciplinary system with a nursing component. The coordinating role of nursing within that interdisciplinary team is well recognized. However, nursing also has a contribution to make because of its specific focus, *the inability of persons to provide the required amount and quality of health-related self-care*. This does not mean that from a self-care deficit nursing theory perspective, nursing is only concerned with individuals.

Nursing is concerned in part with how community variables impact self-care and dependent-care systems and also concerned with intervention at the community level. Examples of community variables that impact self-care include public policies and legislation which contribute to clean air, clean water, a safe food supply, access to transportation, an effective health care system factors, availability and distribution of resources and so on. These variables and their relationships are illustrated in Figure 7.1.

This figure identifies variables associated with a model for nursing practice in the community. On the extreme left hand side of the figure are listed basic conditioning factors which condition the individual variables of self-care, therapeutic self-care demand and self-care agency which appear in the next set of boxes. Some community variables are identified in a separate box. The model suggests that there is a relationship between the basic conditioning factors and the community variables. It also suggests that there is a relationship between the community variables and individual variables. Nurses collect data about the identified variables, exploring relationships and using nursing and related theory to help to attach meaning of this data in reference to the proper object of nursing. This leads to a conclusion about what is. The next step is to identify health outcomes sought or changes required. The health outcomes sought or changes required may be at the level of the individual, at the level of the community, or both. The intervention may be at the level of the individual or at the level of the community. The health outcomes sought and the changes which are possible depend in part on the relationships among the individual variables and the relationship of those variables to the community processes available to bring about desired changes. The processes related

FIGURE 7.1 A Structural Community Nursing Practice Model Derived From Self-Care

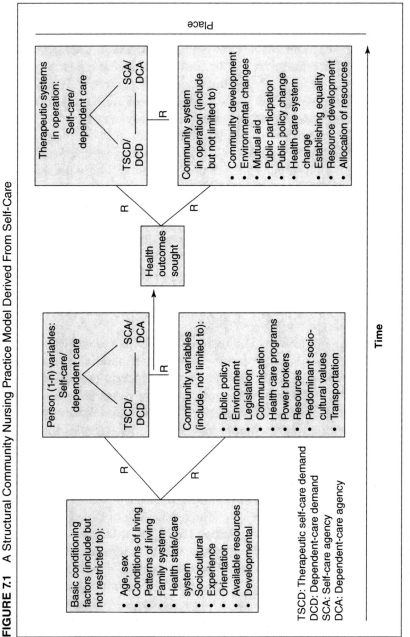

Source: Adapted from S. G. Taylor and K. McLaughlin (1991), "Orem's general theory of nursing and community nursing," *Nursing Science Quarterly, 4,* 153-160.

to the model are described more fully by Taylor and Renpenning (1998) and Taylor and Renpenning in Orem, 2001.

As illustrated in the preceding discussion in addition to nursing being informed by the science of supportive-developmental nursing science, nursing accesses and benefits from related fields—the social sciences, statistics, epidemiology, pathophysiology, bacteriology, education, and others depending on the knowledge base required in the situation in search for an answer to the question, *"what is the relationship between community-related concerns and the provision of the nursing component of the health services?"*

SUMMARY

In this chapter, supportive-developmental nursing science and the manner in which it informs supportive-developmental nursing systems has been discussed. These nursing systems may involve individual persons, dependent-care units, or multiperson units such as communities. Historically, this type of nursing has fallen within the practice of public health or community health nurses. However, with early discharge from acute care facilities and the increasing numbers of nurse practitioners, more and more nurses are involved in supportive-developmental nursing. Establishing a nursing perspective and a nursing theoretical base for these types of nursing systems is essential for determining the nursing contribution and the basis for evidence of nursing practice in primary health care as well as care provided in in-patient settings.

REFERENCES

Artinian, N. T., Magnan, M., Sloan, M., & Lange, M. (2002). Self-care behaviours among patients with heart failure. *Heart and Lung, 31,* 161–172.

Baker, L. K., & Denyes, M. J. (2008). Predictors of self-care in adolescents with cystic fibrosis: A test of Orem's theories of self-care and self-care deficit. *Journal of Pediatric Nursing, 23,* 37.

Carper, B. A. (1978). Fundamental patterns of knowing in nursing. *Advances in Nursing Science, 1,* 13–23.

Dashiff, C. J., McCaleb, A., & Cull, V. (2006). Self-care of young adolescents with type 1 diabetes. *Journal of Pediatric Nursing, 21*(3), 222–232.

Geden, E. A., Taylor, S. G., & Isaramalai, S. (2001). Self-care deficit nursing theory and the nurse: Practitioner's practice in primary care settings. *Nursing Science Quarterly, 14*, 29–33.

Institute of Medicine Committee on the Future of Primary Care. (1996). Defining primary care. In M. Donald, K. Yordy, & N. Vanselow (Eds.), *Primary care: America's health in a new era* (pp. 30–31). Washington, DC: National Academy Press.

Riegel, B., Moser, D. K., Anker, S. D., Appel, L. J., Dunbar, S. B., Grady, K. L., et al. (2009). State of the science: Promoting self-care in persons with heart: A scientific statement from the American Heart Association. *Circulation: Journal of the American Heart Association, 120*, 1141–1163.

Schumacher K. L., Beidler, S. M., Beeber, A. S., Gambino, P. (2006). A transactional model of cancer family caregiving skill. *Advances in Nursing Science, 29*, 271–286.

Schumacher, K. L., Stewart, B. J., Archbold, P. G., Dodd, M. J., & Dibble, S. L. (2000). Family caregiving skill: Development of the concept. *Research in Nursing and Health, 23*, 191–203.

Sochalski, J., Jaarsma, T., Krumholz, H. M., Laramee, A., McMurray, J. J. V., Naylor, M. D., et al. (2009). What works in chronic care management: The case of heart failure. *Health Affairs, 28*, 179–189.

Taylor, S. G., & McLaughlin, K. (1991). Orem's general theory of nursing and community nursing. *Nursing Science Quarterly, 4*, 153–160.

Taylor, S. G., Renpenning, K. M., Geden, E., Neuman, B. M., & Hart, M. A. (2001). A theory of dependent care: A corollary theory to Orem's theory of self-care. *Nursing Science Quarterly, 14*, 39.

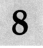

8

Compensatory Nursing Science

PURPOSE AND NATURE OF COMPENSATORY NURSING SCIENCE

Compensatory nursing science is concerned with situations in which persons may have an undeveloped, inoperable, partially operable, or inadequate self-care agency and require the assistance of nursing in the production of the self-care/dependent-care system. The content elements of the science are illustrated in Chapter 6, Figure 6.1. Development of the science occurs with the exploration of these variables in practice situations which require wholly compensatory and partly compensatory nursing systems. The outcome of the development of this science is a basis for understanding evidence in these two types of nursing situations. It connects the foundational nursing sciences with practice and with knowledge available in related disciplines to facilitate understanding of compensatory nursing situations. It also addresses evidence for guiding the interpersonal, societal, and technological operations of nursing, and for the prediction of outcomes associated with compensatory nursing—the basis for evidence-informed nursing decision making and evidence-informed nursing practice.

There are two types of compensatory nursing situations— wholly compensatory and partly compensatory. The nature of the self-care limitations distinguishes wholly compensatory from partly compensatory. The characterizing feature of wholly compensatory nursing situations is the inability of the person to move and perform self-care. This immobility results in a very complex therapeutic self-care demand that is often unstable due to the conditioning effects of the sheer number of factors interacting with each other and with the self-care requisites.

Partly compensatory nursing situations differ from wholly compensatory ones in that the person is able to participate to some degree in production of the self-care system and the impact of mobility on the essential self-care requisites is different. Partly compensatory nursing situations are characterized by persons who have an operable self-care agency but the degree and development for self-management varies depending on the nature and extent of the limitation(s) present. The variations may relate to any one of the components of deliberate action—knowing, decision making, or acting. The situation may be of short term duration such as the period of regaining capability following a surgical procedure to long-term incapacity associated with a chronic illness. Understanding the extent of the limitations and the requirements for nursing begins with calculating the therapeutic self-care demand.

WHOLLY COMPENSATORY NURSING SITUATIONS

The Therapeutic Self-Care Demand

Calculating and meeting the components of the demand in wholly compensatory situations is often an interdisciplinary activity, involving physicians, physiotherapists, nutritionists, respiratory therapists, and so on, in addition to the nurse and the family. It is quite likely that the demand will require frequent and rapid recalculation. The process of calculating the therapeutic self-care demand was described in Chapter 6.

The physiological impact of immobilization on the therapeutic self-care demand and self-care agency may be extensive depending on the cause and the duration of the immobility. Antecedent knowledge that is required to make this impact known includes understanding of the pathophysiology and psychopathology associated with the particular self-care limitations and the effects of the conditioning factors on specific self-care requisites. This makes it possible for nurses to particularize the self-care requisites. At this point in the development of compensatory nursing science, these relationships are in the early stages of being made explicit. The following is offered as an introduction to the utility that pursuing this line of reasoning has for conceptualizing nursing practice in the complex field of compensatory nursing.

Immobility and Essential Self-Care Requisites

When self-care agency is inoperable and the person is not engaging in any form of deliberate action, the impact of immobility is such that there are certain self-care requisites that are always of concern. These have been identified as essential self-care requisites and include

- requisites to maintain life including maintaining an adequate intake of air, food, and water; providing care associated with elimination; maintaining a balance between rest and activity
- requisites to prevent hazards to life, health, and well-being
- requisites to maintain structural and functional integrity including development physically, and mental and emotional normality

In addition, consideration must be given to the regulation or control of distressing symptoms, the regulation or control of stress, ensuring comfort and social contact, and control of environmental factors.

As the relationship between these requisites and the conditioning factors is made explicit, the components of the therapeutic self-care demand are made explicit and provide direction for nursing and for determining the impact of nursing actions—a component of the evidence of the effectiveness of nursing. For example, patients in a coma require artificial feeding—either parenteral or enteral. Although nursing is not in control of prescribing or determining what constitutes a "sufficient intake of food," it is important for nurses to have current knowledge of how this is determined, why it is important, and how to evaluate achievement of meeting this requisite. A "sufficient intake of food" includes neither overfeeding nor underfeeding the patient. Overfeeding or underfeeding have been associated with increased mortality, increased intensive care unit stay, increased infection rates, and decreased rates of spontaneous ventilation (Blackburn, Wollner, & Bistrian, 2010; Ros et al., 2009). The balance is achieved through regulation of volume, caloric intake, nutrients, and methods of administration. The complexity of the impact of the conditioning factors on body functioning, determining the specific purposes to be achieved to meet this requisite is an interdisciplinary activity.

Some examples of the use of the construct therapeutic self-care demand in intensive care nursing are presented. These examples illustrate the utility of the construct in organizing nursing knowledge related to the practice situation, the impact this can have on data included in the patient record, on evidence for practice, and ultimately on the development of nursing practice science. The following discussion is presented as an exemplar neither to be considered complete nor representative of the latest information about each requisite.

The Therapeutic Self-Care Demand and the Data for Evidence

EXAMPLE 1: Concerning the requisite to maintain a sufficient intake of food

Particularizing the Requisite as Part of Determining the Therapeutic Self-Care Demand

If the feeding is to be enteral, a beginning reformulation of the requisite for maintaining an adequate intake of food would include the following:

Maintain an intake of food adequate to

- *reduce threat of malnutrition contributing to loss of lean body mass*
- *maintain the gut barrier*
- *stimulate the immune function*
- *lessen the inflammatory state*
- *support wound healing (Ros et al., 2009)*

The processes for meeting this requisite would include

- *having appropriate feeding available*
- *having specific knowledge of constituents of feeding, potential side-effects, and of the method of administration, for example, anatomy and physiology of the gut, hazards of enteral feeding*
- *performing procedure*
- *evaluating outcomes*

The Data for Evidence

Evidence related to this requisite includes answers to questions such as:

- *Are the orders appropriate?*
- *Do physician and nurse orders reflect use of appropriate protocols?*
- *Is there evidence that the protocols have been followed?*

■ *How much feeding was administered over what period of time?*
■ *Are any identified potential side-effects present?*

Knowing the extent to which this requisite is being met requires links in the patient record to physician orders, nursing orders, protocols regarding enteral feeding, nursing actions, and laboratory data which provides information related to loss of lean body mass, changes in the gut barrier, presence of infection/inflammation.

EXAMPLE 2: Concerning the requisites to maintain a balance between rest and activity and solitude and social interaction

Sleep disturbances in the intensive care unit and intensive care unit delirium are widely reported in the literature. These states impact meeting of the foregoing two requisites. The consequences of deprivation of rapid eye-movement sleep associated with central nervous system depressant medication may be followed by rebound phenomena when there is sudden discontinuance of the medication. This rebound can cause an increase in heart rate, hypoxemia, cardiac arrhythmias, and hemodynamic instability. Figueroa-Ramos, Arroyo-Novoa, Lee, Padilla, and Puntillo (2009) describe some of the consequences of sleep deprivation. These consequences can be addressed in a beginning reformulating of these requisites:

Maintain a balance between rest and activity and solitude and social interaction to prevent

■ *increased pain sensitivity*
■ *reduction in forced expiratory volume*
■ *decreases in parasympathetic cardiac modulation*
■ *impaired immune response*
■ *altered metabolic and endocrine systems*
■ *impaired attention and psychomotor performance*
■ *increased daytime drowsiness*
■ *impaired mood that includes fatigue and irritability*

The Data for Evidence

Evidence related to these requisites includes answers to the following questions.

■ *Are the nursing and physician orders appropriate?*
■ *Is there evidence of action being taken to control the environment, manage pain and discomfort? Is information provided regarding the patient response and the effectiveness of these actions?*

EXAMPLE 3: Concerning regulation or control of stress, ensuring comfort and social contact and control of environmental factors

In studies concerned with patient perceptions of times when wholly compensatory nursing is required, patients report a variety of anxiety producing occurrences and emotions—loneliness, sense of isolation, fears about what is happening to them, humiliation about the way they appear, powerlessness, drifting in and out of reality, disturbed sensory perceptions. A desire for a return to normality is frequently expressed. Interference with sleep is considered to be a factor in exacerbating anxiety. This is only a sampling of an area of concern to nurses working in wholly compensatory nursing. Although the concern is well-substantiated in the literature, there is little reported about specific strategies related to achieving meeting patient need. Controlling the environment is addressed but is almost impossible to achieve without attention to structural and organizational variables. Comforting hands and touch are considered effective strategies by intensive care nurses. Henricson et al. (2009) reported a study in which the use of tactile touch was employed as a means of addressing this component of the therapeutic self-care demand. More research is needed in this area particularly in relation to staff values, education, organizational variables, and effective interpersonal operations in intensive care units. In the meantime, the following are suggested as ways to begin to particularize requisites associated with regulating the physical, biologic, and social environment to prevent development of states of fear, anger, or anxiety.

Particularizing the Requisite

- *Seek understanding of patient/family perception of what is happening*
- *Provide a quiet peaceful environment with periods of light and dark*
- *Organize technical procedures to promote uninterrupted periods of sleep*
- *Establish a consistent pattern of communication with patient recognizing that anger and frustration may be signs of insufficient communication*
- *Provide for continuity of care in assignment of nurses*

The Data for Evidence

Examine staff assignment patterns to determine if continuity of care is being achieved. What information is available regarding extent and quality of sleep time, effective communication strategies, patient/family members concerns, and perceptions of what is happening?

Determining the requirements for meeting these requisites and the role of nurses requires that nurses have access to various components of the patient record and that there is provision for including the pertinent date in the record. This includes but is not limited to the history of the patient's condition; nursing orders, history of nursing action in regard to controlling the environment, facilitating patient comfort, ways in which patient is expressing pain and anxiety, strategies employed to relieve anxiety and patient response, pain management techniques and patient response; the perspective and orders of physicians involved in the situation; data about cardiac function; laboratory data which provides information about the presence of infection, inflammation. If this data can be linked electronically it can be used to analyze cases to determine what works and what doesn't work. Conceptualizing and naming the variables of concern to nursing facilitates this process (Goossen et al., 2004).

Self-Care Limitations and Self-Care Agency

Self-care limitations, introduced in Chapter 3, result in inadequate or inoperable self-care agency. Self-care agency, or the power to produce necessary care is assessed against the required action (the therapeutic self-care demand). The limitations of particular concern in wholly compensatory nursing situations include

- interferences with sensory functioning, perception, memory, and attention deficits that interfere with acquiring or recalling information
- conditions which affect consciousness, cognitive functioning, rational thought processes such as toxic states, mental and emotional illnesses, brain disorders, drug-induced mental and physical disorders
- dispositions and orientations that result in perceptions, meanings, and appraisals of situations that are not in accord with reality
- aberrations in cognitive functioning that affect with knowing when action is to be taken, what action is appropriate, when to stop action, and with organizing a series of actions into meaningful sequences to achieve a particular goal. These limitations may result in a completely inoperable self-care agency as in the unconscious state or extreme mental illnesses. In these situations wholly compensatory nursing systems are indicated. There may also be situations of immobility but the person is able to participate in decision making related to self-care. In these situations a wholly compensatory and a supportive-developmental nursing system would be indicated.

Nursing Systems in Wholly Compensatory Nursing Situations

Designing of nursing systems is carried out by individual nurses caring for individual patients. Designing of nursing systems is also a function of nursing administration in health care organizations. This involves designing care systems for aggregates of patients with common characteristics such as nursing systems for patients with spinal cord injuries, or nursing systems for patients immediately postoperatively (see Allison & Renpenning, 1999, for a detailed explanation of the design function and nursing administration). The nursing system required is a function of the characteristics of the self-care deficit present and the method of helping that is required. The three variations of self-care deficits described give rise to three sub-types of wholly compensatory nursing systems. Each of these variations in turn is associated with particular requirements for variations in the requirements for nursing agency and for the development of nursing knowledge.

Type 1

The first type is concerned with persons who are unable to engage in any form of deliberate action as when a person is in a coma. This includes persons who are unable to control their movement in space, are unresponsive to stimuli, appear unresponsive but who may be responding to stimuli through hearing or feeling, and those who are unable to communicate because of loss of motor ability. In this nursing system, self-care agency is completely inoperable. Some questions to be explored by nursing include the following:

- How does a totally inoperable self-care agency impact the particularization of each of the essential self-care requisites under varying health states?
- How does culture impact the interpersonal dimension and communication in the presence of an inoperable self-care agency? For example, what is the meaning of touch, what kind of touch is or is not appropriate?
- What "end of life" beliefs may be impacting decision making of family members?

Type 2

The second type of wholly compensatory nursing system is concerned with persons who are aware and may be able to make observations and decisions about self-care, but are unable to or should not perform the required actions. In addition to exploring the questions identified in type one, this category of nursing system requires that nurses explore the particular power components for self-care including

■ ability to acquire technical knowledge about self-care from authoritative sources, to retain it, and to operationalize it
■ ability to reason within a self-care frame of reference
■ motivation (i.e., goal orientations for self-care that are in accord with its characteristics and its meaning for life, health, and well-being)

Exploration of the foundational capabilities and dispositions may be appropriate to determine the extent to which persons can and should be encouraged to participate in making observations and decisions about self-care. Also important is determining the validity of the patient contribution and if this is not consistent with the nurse's view, what is the meaning and impact of this discrepancy.

Type 3

The third type of wholly compensatory nursing system is concerned with persons who are unable to attend to themselves and make judgments and decisions about self-care but with continuous guidance and supervision can perform some self-care activities. These persons are unable to focus attention as required for self-care. They may or may not be able to be consistent in making rational judgments and decisions without guidance. They may be ambulatory and able to perform a limited number of self-care operations with supervision. They may need to be protected from hazardous conditions and other persons may need to be protected from them. In these situations it may be helpful to assess the extent to which each of the power components for self-care are operational as this will provide some direction for the extent and nature of the nursing assistance that is required.

In type three situations, it is again important to identify and particularize the essential self-care requisites which are of concern. The impact of variations of conditioning factors on the particularizing of these essential self-care requisites when the above self-care limitations exist make up an important component of knowledge required to effectively deliver nursing services for persons requiring this type of nursing system.

Combinations of Nursing Systems

Supportive educative nursing systems may exist in conjunction with wholly compensatory nursing systems when persons are able to make observations and decisions about self-care but are incapable of acting on their own behalf or should refrain from doing so. It is important that nurses recognize and facilitate patient participation in making decisions as to how and when various components of the self-care demand should be met. For example, in an intensive care unit, although a person may be mechanically ventilated, unable to physically produce self-care, they may still be able to participate in decisions about how they would like to have components of the self-care demand met.

This combination of nursing systems may also be appropriate when self-care and self-management limitations stem from cognitive and emotional states that interfere with self-care operations of knowing, decision-making, or acting; one or more power components for self-care; and/or one or more foundational capabilities and dispositions for deliberate action. Persons may be able to produce the required self-care with guidance, direction, and/or minimal assistance. Persons need assistance in determining what is required and/or support to persist in required activities.

The Theoretical Basis for Wholly Compensatory Nursing Practice

Understandings about the theoretical basis for wholly compensatory nursing practice can be gained by examining the literature in relation to care of patients in intensive care units and in the mental health literature. In wholly compensatory nursing, probably the most significant organizer is the relationship of the basic conditioning factor of health state to self-care requisites. This requires that nurses have an extensive antecedent knowledge about the pathophysiology, psychopathology, and medical treatments of the particular health states of the patient population with which they are concerned so that they can determine the impact of the conditioning effects of these health states on components of the self-care system.

This raises questions about the requirements for educational preparation of nurses working in wholly compensatory nursing situations. The lack of knowledge of a sample of these nurses regarding pulmonary function has been demonstrated (Pirret, 2007). From examination of the knowledge base required for nurses to calculate the therapeutic self-care demand for immobile patients and patients with an inoperable self-care agency it would seem obvious that preparation of nurses is required at least at the master's level and there certainly should be nurses prepared at the doctoral level available in these situations.

Some health states which are most likely to result in the need for a wholly compensatory nursing system include:

- mental health where there are disturbances in cognitive reasoning
- coma or states of unconsciousness
- severe trauma
- postsurgical states
- cases of extreme fatigue
- enforced inoperability of self-care agency

Some of the questions of concern in wholly compensatory nursing science include the following:

- What physiological changes occur in each body system when the body is immobilized or mobility is compromised and how soon do these changes occur?
- What impact does immobility have on the processes of development?
- What/how do nursing actions mitigate the effects of the changes in body systems or the effects on the processes of development?
- What/how do nursing actions unintentionally exacerbate the changes in body systems or the effects of the processes of development?

Wholly compensatory nursing generally takes place in an institution of some kind. This requires nursing to be knowledgeable about how organizational variables can impact nursing practice. This will be considered in detail in Chapter 9. However, consideration of wholly compensatory nursing science is not complete without drawing attention to the importance of exploring the relationship between organizational variables and achieving maximum effectiveness of wholly compensatory nursing.

Nursing Agency

Dawson (2006) suggests that because of the paucity of research to guide the practice of critical care nurses they must become their own researchers choosing appropriate strategies from a variety of options contributing to establishing an evidence base in day-to-day practice. Their practice involves "the dilemma of managing and coordinating the very visible science of critical care technology versus the often invisible art of nursing care" (p. 314). To this, these authors would add often the *invisible component of nursing science*. This can in part be corrected and made visible by naming, recording, and making available information about all of the variables of concern to nursing as facilitated by a nursing practice theory such as self-care deficit nursing theory as well as through continued development of the nursing sciences. This provides the data required. The processes for using that data require that nurses have a clear understanding of the purposes of nursing to enable framing the problem(s) of concern from a nursing perspective. And last, but not least, must have developed the intellectual skills associated with data collection and analysis, as well as being able to evaluate research for evidence-based practice.

The requirements for nursing agency are in part a function of the method of helping. Two methods of helping are predominant in wholly compensatory nursing situations—doing for and providing a supportive-developmental environment. Because the nurse is acting for the patient, the interpersonal component of the nursing system is extremely important. The nature of the relationship that is established with the patient and family impacts the confidence they will have in the nurse's ability. It is only through input from the family and close personal friends that the nurse will be able to initiate knowing the patient as person. The principle of personalism is antecedent to the theories of self-care and dependent care as described in Chapters 1 and 5. The view of the individual as person is foundational to all interpersonal contact nurses have with patients and families. Also of concern in wholly compensatory nursing and within the view of human being as person is the view of human being as object. As object, humans are seen as potentially subject to physical forces over which they have no control and from which they must be protected when they are unable to control their movements in space. The view of human as object is not a depersonalizing view when the view of humans as person is the overarching view subsuming all other views of human beings specific to nursing (Orem, 1997). These views give meaning to one aspect of wholly compensatory nursing—the doing for with the *for* being differentiated as *for* and not *to*.

In nursing situations where persons are unable to communicate their wishes and unable to move their bodies in space, the touch of the nurse has been demonstrated to be a significant nursing intervention. Henricson et al. (2009) suggested that understanding the meaning of tactile touch to the patient can be gained through exploration of the philosophy of ethics formulated by Aristotle. They characterize tactile touch as a caring activity, which occurs slowly over time while time appears to stand still. They demonstrated that while tactile touch was occurring, patients expressed experiencing harmony of mind and body. They suggest exploring Aristotle's view on the nature of human good or human happiness and pleasure can expand understanding of this phenomenon. Understanding the meaning of touch from this perspective is consistent with self-care deficit nursing theory. Unless "knowing nursing" as art as well as technology is considered in developing budgets for intensive care units it is highly unlikely that time for touch being employed in this manner will be included in determining staffing requirements in intensive care units.

PARTLY COMPENSATORY NURSING SITUATIONS

The trends toward limited hospitalization and including family members into caregiving in long-term care settings means preparing the patient and family members for increasing responsibilities to meet immediate care needs, to prevent complications, and to promote healthful living. Self-management capability may be temporarily affected as in the acute phase of an illness or immediately postoperatively. The change in capability may have long-term consequences as in a chronic illness. The changes in capability may give rise to the need for a partly compensatory nursing system.

In the partly compensatory nursing situations, nurses, patients, and possibly family members or other caregivers share in determining the nature of the self-care deficit, the nature of a dependent-care deficit if a dependent-care agent is involved, and in developing and executing the action system required. The culture of the family and health-related beliefs to which a person has been exposed influence choices in relation to self-care actions. Exploring knowledge and beliefs related to the self-care/dependent-care deficit precedes determining how best to help persons achieve self-care goals. Nurse action may include performing some self-care measures for patients, compensating for self-care limitations of patients, or assisting the patient as required in the process of helping them to acquire specific capabilities. Patients will participate in decision-making and choices, perform some self-care measures, regulate self-care agency, dependent-care agents may perform some care measures, and both will accept assistance and care from nurses.

The Therapeutic Self-Care Demand

Again in the following discussion presentation of the specific components of the therapeutic self-care demand is not meant to be complete but only to provide direction for consideration of this component of designing a nursing system.

When a person emerges from the immobility associated with an acute illness, trauma, surgery, and so on the nursing situation changes from one that is wholly compensatory to partly compensatory. As the self-care agency becomes operable the therapeutic self-care demand also changes. These changes are illustrated in the examples which follow.

EXAMPLE 1: Self-care in the immediate postoperative period

In the immediate postoperative period the self-care agency may not be adequate until the effects of the anaesthetic wear off. Until that happens the maintenance of physiological integrity still requires a wholly compensatory nursing system. With return to consciousness the requirements for nursing assistance change depending on the state of cognition and the state of mobility.

The Requisites

During this time the universal self-requisites of concern are:

- *maintaining an adequate intake of air*
- *maintaining an adequate intake of water*
- *prevention of hazards*
- *care regarding processes of elimination*
- *management of pain*

The health deviation self-care requisites of concern would include

- *monitoring for side-effects of any immobility, procedures, medications, other therapies pertinent to specific patient situation.*
- *determining if patient is aware of need for securing assistance, motivated and capable of doing so.*

Strategies for meeting the preceding requisites are addressed in the well-established protocols which are in place in every institution where surgical procedures are carried out. However, components of the therapeutic self-care demand concerned with interpersonal processes and promotion of development are less emphasized. Meeting developmental self-care requisites focuses on "causing no harm" that is establishing an interpersonal relationship which helps to mitigate the unpleasant experiences associated with recovering from a surgical procedure.

The Data for Evidence

The recording of the results of physiological monitoring is adequately addressed in most manual and digital recording systems. Attention needs to be drawn to the need for facilitating recording of the concerns of nursing which address the interpersonal and developmental components of the concerns of nursing.

EXAMPLE 2: The initial rehabilitation phase following a stroke

In the initial time-period immediately following a stroke, the physiological impact of reduced mobility remains a concern and the essential requisites identified as being of concern in wholly compensatory situations still need to be addressed. However, because there is a partially operative self-care agency, the specific purposes to be achieved and related action systems will vary as illustrated in the following examples. Also there are additional requirements to address the issue of evidence of quality nursing practice.

The Requisite Maintaining a Sufficient Intake of Food and Water

Meeting nutritional requirements is now concerned with the amount of food ingested, caloric content, nutritional content, sodium intake, foods to be avoided, consistency of food to accommodate chewing and swallowing difficulties, positioning of person during eating, prevention of constipation and diarrhea, prevention of skin breakdown, personal preferences, providing assistance as required while promoting independence, communication between caregivers about quantity and quality of intake and about personal and interpersonal issues regarding food intake.

Particularizing the Requisites

Maintain sufficient intake of food and water to

- *maintain/achieve desired body weight*
- *meet nutritional requirements*

- *monitor intake of sodium, cholesterol*
- *drink 6–8, six ounce glasses of water daily*

In addition:

- *Position to prevent aspiration and facilitate self-feeding*
- *Allow sufficient time for feeding to ensure adequate intake*

The Data for Evidence

Recording system allows for and facilitates easy recording regarding content and amount of food ingested, progress regarding self-feeding, links to body weight

Particularizing the Requisite

Provision of care associated with elimination

- *adjust dietary intake to prevent constipation/diarrhea*
- *facilitate acceptance of and provide assistance required to maintain hygiene and prevent skin breakdown*

The Data for Evidence

Recording of specific nursing action, condition of the skin.

Particularizing the Requisite

Promotion of solitude and social interaction

- *Preserve energy by providing for frequent uninterrupted rest periods as indicated by patient energy level*
- *Organize nursing activities to achieve monitoring goals with minimal sleep disturbance through the night*

The Data for Evidence

Record of sleep patterns
     Data which will allow for analysis of organization of nursing activities

The Requisites

Promotion of normalcy, overcoming factors which interfere with development, learning to live with the effects of the stroke including establishing a lifestyle that will promote development. There may also be a need to adjust one's self-concept—accepting self as being in a particular state. For example, research related to spinal cord injury has shown it is necessary for the person to accept self as having limitations Paterson and Thorne (2001).

Particularizing the Requisites

Meeting this component of the therapeutic self-care demand is intertwined with the manner of meeting all of the preceding requisites that have been illustrated. This requisite is concerned with the requirement for stroke survivors to cope with the unpredictability and insecurity associated with recovery at the same time as dealing with the changing functional state and emotional lability associated with the stroke. There is a requirement to cope with changes in role execution and relationships that may be temporary or permanent. Of concern are the effects of these changes on family members and close personal friends, and the necessity to cope with the losses accompanying these changes. Communication problems are often superimposed on all of this— mechanical difficulties, temporary or permanent issues related to aphasia, interferences with cognitive processing, communication patterns, and so on. Specific direction for action may include the following:

- *Encourage and allow person to accomplish activities of daily living independently*
- *Seek and accommodate patient preferences in reference to all aspects of care*
- *Encourage discussion about lifestyle changes and impact of role adjustments*
- *Engage in dialogue with family and close personal friends to gain understanding of their perception of the situation, impact on them, impact on relationship with patient from their perspective*

The Data for Evidence

This component of the patient record is an area of "soft" data. It will be descriptive of the perceptions, intuition, and concerns of patient, family members and close personal friends, nurses and other professionals. Specific communication strategies which work and which don't work should be included. Details of patient and family coping strategies, successes, and failures are important. Accessing this data will probably require having some sort of word-search program but if the data is not entered it cannot be retrieved. Including these self-care requisites as part of the overview of nursing is the first step to getting this information into the patient record and available for advancing nursing knowledge and evaluating effectiveness.

Self-Care Limitations and Self-Care Agency

Self-care capabilities are expressions of what a person has learned to do and can do in relation to acquiring knowledge, making decisions, and acting. The self-care limitations are factors which restrict the individual doing what is required currently or as a result of changing circumstances. Knowing the nature of the self-care limitation, the cause of it, and the expected duration influence the choice of method of helping and the design of the nursing system. The significance of determining self-care limitations and recording data in the patient record about them is illustrated in the following example.

A patient is hospitalized because of severe respiratory distress. Her color is good but there is evidence of consolidation in the lower lobes of both lungs and she has severe sharp right-sided pain. On admission 300 ml of fluid are aspirated from the right chest. She is diagnosed with pneumonia, congestive heart failure is ruled out, and she is treated with antibiotics, an intravenous prednisone preparation, and a diuretic. Her symptoms subside and she is discharged in 5 days. She interprets the investigation of her cardiac status as evidence that her heart is weak from coughing. She is sent home on antibiotics and a diuretic. She complains that the "water pill" is upsetting her stomach— "they always do" and she thinks it is not doing any good as she is not voiding any more than usual. She thinks it is just causing her to have really bad night sweats. Although she was instructed to drink six-eight glasses of water with the antibiotic, she has decided to cut back on her drinking since she's on the water pill. She doesn't take her antibiotic every day. Two weeks later she is again very short of breath and coughing more. Her doctor wants to readmit her to hospital and have her seen by a respirologist. She does not want to go. She does not want to be poked anymore and she does not think they did anything for her the last time. In previous health-related episodes, she has chosen to follow the instructions of a naturopath rather than a physician.

Analysis of the above scenario from the perspective of self-care limitations is interesting. There is a requirement for the patient to do things differently—take medication. Her understanding of how, when, and why of the medication regime, her understanding of bodily functions, and her basic distrust of the medical system are limitations which are interfering with the knowledge acquisition, decision making, and action. No one in the health-care system appears to be aware of the presence of these limitations. The patient had been given written instructions about the medications. Had the area of self-care limitations been explored, preparation for the patient to return home would have been quite different.

In addition to determining self-care limitations and their potential impact, the diagnostic process associated with self-care agency includes assessing capability against the current therapeutic self-care demand to determine the self-care deficit.

The Nursing System

In the partly compensatory nursing system, nurses, patients, and possibly family members or other caregivers share in determining the nature of the self-care deficit, the nature of dependent-care deficit if a dependent-care agent is involved, and developing and executing the action system required. The culture of the family and health-related beliefs to which a person has been exposed influence choices in relation to self-care actions. Exploring knowledge and beliefs related to the self-care/dependent-care deficit precedes determining how best to help persons achieve self-care goals. Nursing action may include performing some self-care measures for patients, addressing self-care limitations of patients, or assisting the patients as required in the process of helping them to acquire specific capabilities. Patients will participate in decision-making and choices, perform some self-care measures, regulate self-care agency. Dependent-care agents may perform some care measures. Both self and dependent-care agents will accept help from nurses. Questions to be considered in designing the nursing system include the following:

Is the developmental state of this person such that it is reasonable to expect that a person will have or be able to acquire the related knowledge and skill?

Is the developmental state such that it can be expected that the person will persist in the necessary activities?

Is there evidence that the person has the required cognitive capacity to make the necessary changes to the self-care system?

Does the person have sufficient energy to devote to self-care?

Is the person motivated to persist in the required activity?

Are there family system factors which will facilitate or interfere with carrying through with the required self-care system? What if any action is appropriate regarding the interferences?

Are there adequate resources available or can these be made available?

COMPENSATORY NURSING SITUATIONS AND DEPENDENT CARE

A dependent-care system may also be involved in partly compensatory nursing situations. The theory of dependent care (Chapter 5) provides a structure, direction for exploring this type of nursing situation and helping nurses to understand this complex situation. The dependent care may involve family members assisting in the care of children or other family members in acute-care settings, in the home, and frequently in long-term care settings.

The dependent-care unit is made up of the person requiring assistance and the caregiver(s). The variables of concern include the therapeutic self-care demand, self-care agency, and self-care deficit of the dependent person, the dependent-care demand, the self-care system of the dependent-care agent, and dependent-care agency of the caregiver. If there is more than one dependent-care agent involved, the dependent-care system becomes more complicated as the variations in dependent-care agency and self-care system of each caregiver and the interactions between caregivers must be considered. Also of concern is the impact on the dependent person of the variations that each dependent-care giver brings to the system. In addition, if there is a nurse involved, then nursing agency must also be considered. These variables and their interrelationships are illustrated in Figure 8.1.

The Nursing System

The nursing system in dependent-care situations is very complex. It helps if one clearly separates two constructs—dependent-care unit (the persons) and dependent-care/nursing system (the actions). The characteristics of the nursing system are a function of the characteristics of the persons making up the dependent-care unit and the dependent-care deficit, which is a description of the relationship between the self-care deficit of the dependent and the capabilities of the caregiver(s). The nursing system may be a supportive-developmental system focusing on development of the capabilities of the caregiver. It may also include a compensatory component to address components of the self-care deficit of the dependent.

The length of time that a dependent-care system will be required is an important consideration. If it is a short-term situation, such as during the postoperative period, in-depth analysis may not be necessary. But if the system is going to be required on an on-going basis, a thorough

FIGURE 8.1   Elements of a Nursing System in Dependent-Care Situations

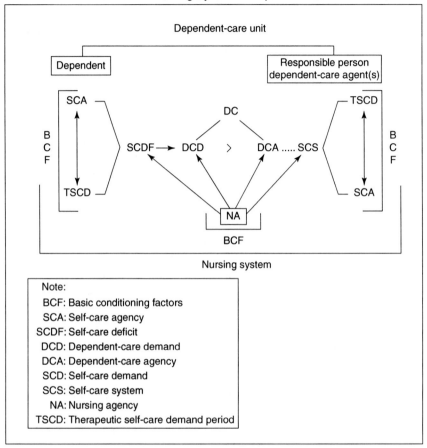

Note:
BCF: Basic conditioning factors
SCA: Self-care agency
SCDF: Self-care deficit
DCD: Dependent-care demand
DCA: Dependent-care agency
SCD: Self-care demand
SCS: Self-care system
NA: Nursing agency
TSCD: Therapeutic self-care demand period

evaluation early may prevent future difficulties. Part of the on-going assessment and design processes related to dependent-care systems include not only evaluating if the caregivers have the capabilities currently required to provide the assistance needed, but also building in a process for acquiring skills that may be required in response to changes in the therapeutic self-care demand. Does the dependent-care agent and/or patient know what to watch for, what to do, when to do something, and when to call for help? Based on the conditioning factors present, it may be possible to anticipate the caregiving trajectory and plan for this, not only in relation to knowledge and skill acquisition for the immediate situation, but also acquiring capabilities associated with recognizing the changes in the therapeutic self-care demand of the dependent which may occur over time and responding to these changes.

In the initial stages of dependent care, the dependent-care agent is required to not only acquire skills related to the caregiving role, but must adjust their self-care system to incorporate the new caregiving requirements while still meeting their own self-care needs. Exploration by nursing into this area may be helpful in preventing future difficulties in accommodating both roles.

The social-interpersonal dimension of the dependent-care system

Dependent care is produced in a dyadic relationship. From the perspective of the dependent-person, that dyadic relationship changes with each new caregiver. Not only does each caregiver "have their own way of doing things" within the technological component of the care system, but the interpersonal relationship is different with each caregiver. If the caregiving situation is going to persist over time, this can become a significant variable in determining the success of the caregiving process especially from the perspective of the dependent person.

Consideration must be given to the nature of the relationship between the dependent and dependent-care agent. Some of the factors to consider include the following:

■ Is it a close personal relationship?
■ Is it a "stormy" relationship?
■ Are both parties agreeable to a dependent-care system and all that it implies?
■ If physical contact is required, how does each person in the relationship feel about that—does the dependent-care agent have health-related issues that may impact on dependent-care agency?
■ Does the dependent-care agent have sufficient energy and willingness to persist in the required dependent care?

Diagnostic operations and the dependent-care agency

The reason for a dependent-care system is the self-care deficit of the dependent person. Diagnosing capability to provide dependent care involves exploration of dependent-care limitations and the relationship between dependent-care agency and dependent-care demand.

Dependent-care agency develops in response to the need of another for assistance in their health-related self-care. The skills required relate to being able to anticipate and recognize changes in the therapeutic self-care demand of the dependent, coping with those changes emotionally, and having a skill repertoire to take appropriate action, as well as performing caregiving activities which have been predefined. Dependent-care limitations may in part be a reflection of any self-care limitations of a caregiver. For example, if the caregiver has limited understanding of how their own body functions, that limited understanding will be reflected in decisions made and actions taken in the caregiving situation. Consequently, the nurse must be aware of the self-care limitations of the caregiver and the impact these limitations may have on the caregiving process as well as identifying dependent-care limitations.

The diagnostic processes associated with the dependent-care agency also determine the stage of development, adequacy, and operability of dependent-care capabilities in relation to the current self-care deficit. It may also include determining the capability of the dependent-care agent to identify and respond to changes in the therapeutic self-care demand and self-care agency of the dependent. As with self-care agency there are factors which condition the dependent-care agency. These include the severity of the illness, the complexity of the technology required, the intensity of the dependent's suffering, the care agents' tolerance for being involved in the care of another (Taylor et al., 2001).

Taylor and Robinson-Purdy (1989) studied the processes of assessing self-management and dependent-care capabilities of hospitalized adults and caregivers in preparation for discharge. Geden and Taylor (1999) described the collaborative system of couples in a dependent-care situation. These works, with additional input from literature related to caregivers, have resulted in development of a screening tool (Exhibit 8.1) which can be useful in assessing patients and families in preparation for discharge from hospital.

The theoretical basis for nursing in situations involving caring for a dependent family member is primarily addressed in literature associated with caregiving. In reading the literature associated with caregiving there appear to be significant gaps concerning both the caregiver and the recipient, including a theoretical framework for exploring the totality of these complex nursing situations. The literature addresses caregiver burden, the processes related to caregiving, and the need for caregiver skill. However, as in nursing process when nursing theory is absent, the content and reasons for developing specific caregiving capabilities and executing specific caregiving actions is missing. The theory of dependent care provides guidance not only in identifying variables but in naming them. For example, introducing the concept

EXHIBIT 8.1
Data Items to Be Considered in Evaluation of Dependent-Care Situation

A. Patient variables
   a. Willingness to have each potential caregiver involved
   b. Performance of activities of daily living
   c. Ability to work with body
   d. Cognitive ability
   e. Compliance level
   f. General health state
   g. Emotional stability
   h. Level of anxiety
   i. Level of energy
   j. Presence of symptoms
   k. Motivation
B. Primary caregiver factors (Dependent-care agent)
   a. Past experiences with caregiving
   b. Impaired mental processes
   c. Motivation to care for another
   d. Cognitive ability
   e. Physical limitations
   f. General health state
   g. Ability to work with another's body
   h. Emotional stability
   i. Level of anxiety
   j. Level of energy
C. Home environment factors
   a. Safety issues re: caregiving at home
   b. Access to support by other persons or agencies
   c. Facilities for privacy
   d. Access to needed equipment, supplies
D. Demand (task) related factors
   a. Need for manipulation of special equipment
   b. Complexity of tasks
   c. Critical observations needed
   d. Expected duration of tasks
   e. Number of activities necessary
   f. Amount of coordination of activities
   g. Amount of equipment needed
E. Additional areas to be explored
   a. Impact of caregiving situation on family functioning
   b. Congruence between patient and caregiver re care required

Source: Adapted from Taylor, S.G. & Robinson-Purdy, V. *Assessing self-management and dependent-care capabilities of hospitalized adults and care givers in preparation for discharge.* Unpublished paper.

of dependent-care demand, which is derived from analysis of the relationship between therapeutic self-care demand and self-care agency of the dependent, helps to address these deficiencies. This content, the focus of the caregiving action, forms the basis for determining the dependent-care demand—"the summations of care measures at a specific point in time or over a duration of time for meeting the dependent's therapeutic self-care demand when his or her self-care agency is not adequate or operational" (Taylor et al., 2001, p. 40). This provides the basis for identifying the knowledge and skill required for caregiving situations, gives direction for understanding the context in which the care is provided, and the impact of that context on the skills and processes involved.

In studies related to family caregivers of persons with cancer, Schumacher et al. (2000) describe the development of the concept *family caregiving skill* identifying that some caregivers "do" caregiving better than others and address the need for nurses to identify what factors make the difference. These authors go on to address the need to understand this process better so that tools can be developed which would assist nurses to asses caregiving skill.

The construct of caregiving skill was subsequently reconceptualized as caregiver skill (Schumacher, 2006). This reconceptualization changed the focus of attention from the person providing the care to the processes associated with the care. The reconceptualization was not based in a nursing theory. Ultimately, in the process of data analysis, the researchers defined family caregiving as a "process that occurs in response to an illness and encompasses multiple cognitive, behavioral, and interpersonal processes." Caregiving skill was defined as "the ability to respond effectively and smoothly to the demands of the illness and pattern of care using these processes." This incorporation of demands of the illness situation and the interaction between the demands arising from the illness and the requirement for care is consistent with the basic understandings associated with the theory of dependent care—specifically the construct of dependent-care demand and understanding that caregiving occurs within an interpersonal frame of reference which influences not only the actions required but the results of those actions. However, the missing piece, still to be formalized by nursing science is the detail related to the therapeutic self-care demand of persons receiving treatment for cancer and for assessment of family "caregiving skills."

In the meantime, self-care deficit nursing theory provides direction for development of discharge instructions for persons with cancer and for their caregivers. The caregiving processes that have been iden-tified in the literature include monitoring, interpreting, making deci-sions, taking action, making adjustments. The content associated with those processes can be determined by linking the conditioning effects of the cancer treatment with the self-care requisites affected by the spe-cific treatment. In general, treatment for cancer impacts the following requisites:

- Maintaining a sufficient intake of food and water
- Maintaining a balance between rest and activity and solitude and social interaction
- Preventing hazards
- Promoting normalcy
- Overcoming factors which interfere with development
- Securing medical assistance
- Being aware of and attending to pathologic conditions and states
- Carrying out diagnostic, therapeutic, and rehabilitation measures
- Attending to comfort
- Modifying self-concept
- Modifying lifestyle

Specifying the content for these processes involves the following:

- Determining the conditioning effect of various treatments for spe-cific forms of cancer on specific self-care requisites
- Developing specific goals to be achieved for these requisites, for ex-ample, maintaining a sufficient intake of food, monitoring for dete-rioration in condition, reporting significant changes to appropriate person
- Specifying how this will be achieved—provide diet with specific ca-loric intake of required consistency, monitor daily intake, and keep a record of days when person does not eat, check weight weekly, report to physician/nurse if weight loss has exceeded three pounds
- Evaluating caregivers capability in reference to the specifications of the actions required—do they understand importance of monitor-ing weight, are they likely to do this, does the family have a scale, do they know who to contact regarding changes

The difference that self-care deficit nursing theory makes in the above situation is the direction for identifying content to achieve the required self-care/dependent care—what is required, the action system to achieve what is required, evaluating capability for achieving or producing the required actions. There is also direction for evaluating the extent to which the goals are being achieved and the effectiveness of nursing involvement.

MODELS OF NURSING CASES

Improvement of nursing practice is in part dependent on our ability to study cases, look for commonalities, theorize about best practices in relation to those commonalities, establish theoretical basis for suggested practices, and judge the efficacy of those practices. The outcome of these activities is development of a nursing science knowledge base about components of nursing practice with common characteristics which enable us to develop models for a variety of purposes. Determining types of nursing cases for the purposes of developing models and rules of practice involves analyzing nursing cases, identifying variables which can be used as organizers, looking for recurrence of relationships among those variables, and describing patterns of occurrence. This data can be used to identify nursing cases with like characteristics enabling nursing to develop models which provide direction for developing rules of practice for nursing—"when conditions *abc* are present in a situation, the preferable nursing action is *xyz*."

Early in the development of self-care deficit nursing theory, the Nursing Development Conference Group (Nursing Development Conference Group [NDCG], 1979) developed a descriptive model of the variables associated in the stages of a cerebral vascular accident which is an exemplar of organizing information for one category of nursing cases. This model has been helpful to nurses in developing an understanding of what is meant by conceptualizing nursing variables from a population perspective and constructing a model representative of requirements for nursing. An extract of this model is presented as an exemplar. In this model, the interrelationship of the variables therapeutic self-care demand, self-care agency, and nursing agency for two stages of cerebrovascular accident is illustrated (Table 8.1).

This is not meant as an up-to-date or complete presentation or organization of current knowledge related to this population. Note the term "requirements" is used. This term preceded the use of "requisite." Also, this work precedes formalization of the concepts of developmental self-care requisites and dependent care.

TABLE 8.1
A Descriptive Model of Nursing System Variables

ACUTE STAGE OF CEREBROVASCULAR ACCIDENT	
A. Unconscious Phase of Severe Stroke	B. Phase of Returning Consciousness
Population	*Population*
Persons who have had a severe stroke recently	Individuals who recently sustained a stroke and who are not yet medically stable but are regaining consciousness
Types of Self-Care Limitations	*Components of Therapeutic Self-Demand*
Lack of awareness of environment and inoperative mental processes	Self-monitoring and universal self-care modifications still required as in Stage II A with reemergence of the need to be normal
Inoperative protective reflexes	Reorientation of self to persons, places, things in environment
Immobility (with its range of hazards to the structural and functional integrity of the organism)	Acknowledgment of changes in self
Composition of the Therapeutic Self-Care Demand	Reestablishment of communication systems
Modification of entire range of universal self-care requirements	Beginning resumption of aspects of integrated human functioning requisite to self-care agency (e.g., decision-making)
Frequent monitoring of multiple physiologic variables	Cooperation with performance of measures of care associated with the therapeutic modalities
Administration and monitoring of effects of specific drugs (e.g., antihypertensives, anticoagulants)	Avoiding activities that may increase intracranial pressure
Detection and management of life-threatening complications	Extensive deficit for engagement in self-care due to the stroke. Extent of self-care deficit varies with severity of the stroke.
Self-care agency may not be operative in persons who have had severe strokes, and the deficit for engagement in self-care will be complete qualitatively and quantitatively.	

Components of Nursing Agency	Types of Self-Care Agency Limitations
Theoretical knowledge of	Mental confusion, memory gaps, and/or emotional lability (that will impair judgment and decision-making)
—pathophysiology of stroke	Denial of paralysis; neglect of affected side
—normal parameters and interrelationships of variables reflecting health state; deviations from the norm that require immediate referral and action	Some combination of sensory, perceptual, motor, and communication impairments
—effects and consequences of immobility	
—causes and effects of unconscious state	Theoretical Knowledge
—rationale for and therapeutic and untoward effects of medical treatment modalities	—all types required for Stage II A plus
—crisis and crisis intervention theory	—usual patterns of recovery from stroke and of return to conscious state
Skills for or in the nature of	—theory concerning human sensation, perceptual, cognitive, emotional, memory, emotion, motivation; body—and self-image, experience of loss, and stages of grieving process
—techniques for meeting universal self-care requirements (to maintain circulation and oxygenation of tissues, nutrition and fluid balance, musculoskeletal integrity, skin and mucous membrane integrity, elimination, a balance of rest and sensory social stimulation, and safety of environment) in unconscious individual	—major types of sensory, perceptual, cognitive, emotional, motor deficits that occur following stroke
—assessment of family's level of coping	Skills
—crisis intervention techniques	—all types required for Stage A plus
—assessment of neurological status and other body systems reflecting health state	—assessment of signs or returning consciousness and types and severity of deficits for action

(Continued)

TABLE 8.1 (*Continued*)

ACUTE STAGE OF CEREBROVASCULAR ACCIDENT	
—administration of special treatment modalities	—reorientation and remotivation techniques
—recognition of condition changes that indicate life-threatening emergencies and require immediate intervention or referral	—assessment of signs of readiness to participate in self-care and/or contraindications to increasing participation
—designing, operationalizing, and managing complex wholly compensatory nursing systems through which the universal and health deviation self-care requirements within therapeutic self-care demand are integrated and met through nurse actions.	—establishment of communication systems and supportive interpersonal environments

Source: An excerpt from NDCG, 1979. Used with permission.

SUMMARY

In this chapter the elements of the nursing sciences that inform wholly and partly compensatory nursing situations have been presented. The discussion of nursing cases and theoretical understandings is a beginning. It has been illustrated how continuing study of such nursing situations within a nursing theoretical framework can facilitate ongoing understanding of the basis or nursing practice, the development of nursing science, and ultimately lead to evidence-informed decision-making and evidence-based nursing practice.

REFERENCES

Allison, S. A., & McLaughlin-Renpenning, K. (1999). *Administration in the 21st century: A self-care theory approach.* Thousand Oaks, CA. Sage Publications.

Blackburn, G. L., Wollner, S., & Bistrian, B. R. (2010). Nutrition support in the intensive care unit: An evolving science. *Archives of Surgery, 145,* 533–538.

Dawson, D. (2006). The art of nursing: A hidden science? *Intensive and Critical Care Nursing, 22,* 313–314.

Figueroa-Ramos, M. I., Arroyo-Novoa, C. M., Lee, K. A., Padilla, G., & Puntillo, K. A. (2009). Sleep and delirium in ICU patients: A review of mechanisms and manifestations. *Intensive Care Medicine, 35,* 781–795.

Geden, E. A., & Taylor, S. G. (1999). Theoretical and empirical description of adult couples' collaborative self-care systems. *Nursing Science Quarterly, 12,* 329–334.

Goossen, W. T. F., Ozbolt, J. G., Goenen, A., Park, H., Mean, C., Einfors, M., et al. (2004). Development of a provisional domain model for nursing process for use within the health level 7 reference information model. *Journal of the American Medical Informatics Association, 11,* 186–194.

Henricson, M., Segesten, K., Berglund, A., & Määttä, S. (2009). Enjoying tactile touch and gaining hope when being cared for in intensive care—a phenomenological hermeneutical study. *Intensive and Critical Care Nursing, 25,* 323–331.

Nursing Development Conference Group. (1979). In D. E. Orem (Ed.), *Concept formalization in nursing: Process and product* (2nd ed., pp. 258–265). Boston: Little, Brown. Copyright Orem Estate.

Orem, D. E. (1997). Views of human beings specific to nursing. *Nursing Science Quarterly, 10,* 26–31.

Paterson, B. L., & Thorne, S. (2001). Critical analysis of everyday self-care decision making in chronic illness. *Journal of Advanced Nursing, 335*–341.

Pirret, A. M. (2007).The level of knowledge of respiratory physiology articulated by intensive care nurses to provide rationale for their clinical decision-making. *Intensive Critical Care Nursing, 23,* 145–155.

Ros, C., McNeill, L., & Bennett, P. (2009). Review: Nurses can improve patient nutrition in intensive care. *Journal of Clinical Nursing, 18,* 2406–2415.

Schumacher, K.L., Beidler, S. M., Song, A., Beeber, A. S., & Gambino, P. (2000). A transactional model of cancer family caregiving skill. *Advances in Nursing Science, 29,* 271–286.

Schumacher, K. L., Stewart, B. J., Archbold, P. G., Dodd, M. J., & Dibble, S. L. (2000). Family caregiving skill: Development of the concept. *Research in Nursing & Health, 23,* 191–203.

Taylor, S. G., Renpenning, K. E., Geden, E. A., Neuman, B. M., & Hart, M. A., (2001). A theory of dependent-care: A corollary theory to orem's theory of self-care, *Nursing Science Quarterly, 14,* 39–47.

Taylor, S. G., & Robinson-Purdy, A. V. (1989, October). *Assessing self-management and capabilities of hospitalized adults and care givers in preparation for discharge.* Paper presented at the first international Self-Care Deficit Nursing Theory Conference, University of Missouri–Columbia, Kansas City.

9

The Science of Self-Care and Evidence-Based Nursing Practice

*T*here are two reasons for developing nursing science and knowledge. One is to improve the profession of nursing—the place of professional nursing in the broader world of health care and human services. The other and more important reason is for the betterment of the persons receiving nursing services, be these individuals, families, communities. The ultimate goal of knowledge development in a profession is that it be translated into practical knowledge. The journey from inspiration, creative thinking, or speculation to practice can be long and circuitous. How knowledge will be used may be logically proposed or thought about but not known at the start of its development and sometimes it remains unknown only to become practical when joined with some other piece of knowledge at some future time. Like creating a mosaic, the design only comes into view when enough pieces are in place. Each piece is important; the sooner it can be connected to the overall structure the more it will contribute to the whole. The development of the mosaic of nursing occurs with each piece of evidence discovered through the several modes of knowledge development—the science of nursing, the art of nursing, personal knowledge, and the moral component (Carper, 1978). Each contributes to the overall body of nursing knowledge when connected to the structure of the discipline of nursing and professional practice.

Structure suggests a framework, overall design, matrices of concepts, middle-range theories, discrete pieces of knowledge, all coming together over time. The types of knowledge and science used in building the structure that is the discipline of nursing and professional practice was introduced in Chapter 1. This is the beginning of building evidence to guide practice. Knowledge developments in the practice setting are also a component of the evidence required for practice. Science informs practice but practice requires development and validation in the real world of patient/client care and the diffusion of innovations to the broader community of nurses. Although there is a concern for translation of theory to practice, the converse is also important. Findings generated from practice need to be connected to our theoretical understanding of the sciences of nursing.

Nursing services are designed and produced for individuals, groups of persons or populations with specific requirements for nursing. Provision of health-related services occurs within a specific political and socio-economic environment influenced by a world-wide perspective on health services. This has resulted in the perception that evidence-based practice is one way of providing the best available cost-effective service to most people. But what is "evidence" in relation to nursing, the service of interest?

DEFINING EVIDENCE

As strange as it may seem there are many ways to define evidence. Evidence may be viewed colloquially as "anything that establishes a fact or gives reason for believing something" (Lomas, Culyer, McCutcheon, McAuley, & Law, 2005, p. 1). Relevance becomes key. Colloquial evidence includes evidence about resources, professional judgment, situational contingencies, and similar factors. Researchers view evidence scientifically as "the use of systematic, replicable methods for production" (Lomas et al., 2005, p. 1) developed through methodologies acceptable to the scientific discipline. However, it becomes more complicated. Lomas goes on to describe two approaches to scientific evidence. One views evidence as context free as in evidence-based medicine. The other allows evidence to be context-sensitive as in the view of the social sciences. So there are in essence three broad conceptualizations for evidence. Each serves a different purpose. Nursing situations are very seldom context free so the colloquial view and that tending toward the social science perspective are generally more useful for nursing. The complexity of health-related situations is illustrated in the following:

> Evidence of the optimal combination of agents to treat Alzheimer's disease would require 127 randomized controlled trials, 63,500 patients and 286 years. (Upshur, 2002, p. 117)

Dictionary definitions of evidence include something that makes another thing evident, indication, sign; something that tends to prove, grounds for belief; law—establishes a point—distinguished from testimony and proof. So evidence establishes a point, or grounds for belief, it is testimony, but it is not proof. It can be inferred from this definition that choice, perception, time, and change are among the elements inherent in the term evidence. Translating this to design and delivery of a health-related service, determining what is best available and most cost-effective entails making choices among competing agendas at the level of the individual practitioner, the organization providing the service, the policy developers, and the provider of the funding for the service. What is the purpose of the evidence? Is it to make economic decisions? Is it to make clinical decisions? And if clinical, what are the boundaries and parameters of the professional service?

Adding to this conundrum is that making wise choices is dependent on having access to data which will inform those decisions. Some of that data comes from specific research. Some comes from data collected as a by-product of the interaction between the professional and the person being served. The data collection and analysis process is complex when the data is numerical but access to digital records has improved the ability to manage and retrieve numerical data. The process of collecting, retrieving, and analyzing data that is not numerical is a challenge. Even more challenging for nursing is capturing and naming the data elements that are involved in nursing decision making. Still to be determined for many nurses is the answer to the question "what is the concern of nursing?"

Early in its development, the role of nurses in hospital-based practice was supportive to the physician's role. Education of nurses improved, questions were raised about the purposes of nursing. Conceptual models for nursing practice and related theories were developed. Nurses in practice began to be able to express what they were about. Advanced practice nurses came on the scene. The predominant model guiding practice for the advanced practice nurse is the medical model, not a nursing model. Geden et al. (2001) described the difference in advanced practice when a nursing model is used. They describe the focus of nursing as the self-care practices of the patient/client and the differences in service provided by nursing with that as the focus. The explicit and tacit models which nurses use to frame their thinking and their practice has meaning for defining what constitutes evidence in nursing practice.

The lack of a clear focus for nursing and a language to describe that focus and the variables associated with nursing has resulted in nursing using what could be termed "surrogate" information to determine effectiveness of a service. This is reflected in using incidence of medication errors, medication compliance, pressure sores, and number of falls as measures of quality services. This is similar to an incident at a border crossing when the immigration officer asked to see the person's passport or birth certificate as proof of citizenship. A driver's license was offered in lieu of that information. The immigration officer said "This doesn't tell me anything. It only tells me you can drive a car." Similarly, with the information about incidence of pressure sores and number of falls—it only tells us how many pressure sores and how many falls.

So what is evidence-informed nursing decision making and evidence-based nursing and how do we achieve it? There are two theoretical bases involved: the theoretical base underlying the nursing component and the theoretical base underlying knowledge translation.

The Theoretical Base Underlying the Nursing Component of Evidence-Based Practice

In *Introduction to Evidence-Based Practice in Nursing and Health Care*, Porter-O'Grady identifies the first step in developing evidence-based practice in the statement, "each discipline must clearly define its specific and unique accountability for clinical decision making, clinical action, and interdisciplinary interaction" (Porter-O'Grady, 2010, p. 16). In Chapter 1 the *proper object* of the discipline of nursing was established as *the inability of a person to provide for self or their dependent child the quality and quantity of health-related self-care that is required*. The continuum through which nursing knowledge is developed is the foundation for consideration of evidence-informed nursing decision making and evidence-based nursing practice.

The stages of understanding nursing begin with the study of nursing cases and situations of nursing practice. This leads to development of a general theory of nursing practice, to the development of related foundational nursing sciences and the nursing practice sciences, to the need for integration of these theoretical components with practice derived knowledge. Each of these topics are discussed in detail in the ensuing chapters.

The proper object of nursing provides direction for making specific the domain, boundaries, and role of nursing in the interdisciplinary health care services. The role of nursing includes individual nurses designing and implementing nursing systems for individual clients, dependent-care units, and families. It includes nurses in management roles designing and facilitating implementation of nursing services for populations of concern to nursing. It includes the role of nursing administration and researchers making known the links between patient health care needs, nursing resources, and the nursing care processes within the context of the health care system, and the social, political, and cultural environments of care. Accepting the proper object of the discipline as described, evidence-based nursing can be defined as:

> *The design, production, and control of nursing systems and the nursing component of interdisciplinary patient care services based on the best available understanding of the sciences and research underlying nursing practice, integrated with the interpersonal, sociopolitical, and economic context of the situation.*

Knowledge development precedes knowledge translation. Knowledge development within a practice discipline such as nursing is dependent on input from practitioners as well as that of academic scholars. Much of nursing practice occurs within health care organizations. Consequently the organization has a strong influence on the focus of nursing activity and the course that knowledge development will take. This development must be valued within the organization and strategies must be in place for the processes related to knowledge development to occur.

The focus of Section II of this book is on the structure and development of the related disciplinary sciences which inform nursing practice—the sciences of wholly compensatory, partly compensatory, and supportive-educative nursing. These sciences are in the early stages of their development. The development of these sciences includes collecting data about nursing cases, analyzing that data, identifying patterns of relationships, developing and validating models and rules of practice. The underlying key to these activities is access to meaningful data that allows for manipulation, integration, and development of new understandings. Some of this can take place in a research environment, but how much more useful and economical it would be if it could take place as a component of the day-to-day activities of clinical practice. Continuing knowledge development is dependent on reflective practitioners and scholars working together in research endeavors and practice, and the feedback loop that is fostered between theory, research, and practice in the exchange of new understandings and building on shared knowledge.

The Theoretical Base Underlying the Knowledge Translation Component of Evidence-Based Practice

We live in a rapidly changing world with a knowledge explosion that organizations concerned with delivering health care services are challenged to make available to professionals for the benefit of their clients. *Unless the administration of the health service entity understands and values the knowledge translation process, how it occurs, the impediments to it happening, and the role it plays in evidence-based nursing, there can be little or no evidence-based practice.*

Much has been written about how nurses access and use information to guide practice. In an extensive review of the current literature, Spenceley, O'Leary, Chizawsky, Ross, and Estabrooks, (2008) confirmed the "predominant use of informal, interactive sources of knowledge, and the influence of contextual factors such as role expectations and assumptions about information-seeking to support practice" (pp. 966–977). Nurses most frequently appeared to use human sources of information. Within the context of scarce resources, nurses are being required to do more with less. Information science literature would direct the health care industry to look to the link between knowledge requirements and the information systems. Embedding best practice guidelines in those systems can be helpful. Capturing the knowledge base of reflective nursing practitioners is essential.

Reflective practitioners are persons who have established a life-long learning attitude toward their own clinical practice. They engage regularly in thinking about, analyzing, and reflecting on the clinical situations they encounter, stay up-to-date on the current literature relative to their practice and endeavor to employ the best strategies that they know of to bring about safe and effective patient care. All nurses should be encouraged to be reflective practitioners. To be reflective practitioners, nurses need access to data they have collected. Not only do they need to be able to access this data but it must be available to them in an easily retrievable form allowing for manipulation of that data to gain insight into relationships among the elements. How can this be accomplished? For the most part, nurses do not keep private patient records. These records are kept within the employing institution. In addition, because nurses practice primarily within some kind of organizational structure rather than as individual practitioners, health care organizations become major players in the focus of the practicing nurse, in the kind of data collected by nurses, in how that data is stored, and ultimately in the development of nursing knowledge. With the decline in emphasis on theory-based practice, the evidence-based practice movement is like a ship at sea without a rudder.

For years, medicine has conducted regular chart reviews—accessing records using diagnoses on admission and/or discharge, and discharge summaries. The medical records, reasons for admission, and discharge summaries include data items that are reflective of the concerns of medicine. By doing these chart reviews, medicine has built up a knowledge base, developed diagnostic categories, and provided opportunities for practitioners to expand their knowledge base. Medicine was seen by the funders of health care organizations as being the driving force behind cost. Thus, diagnostic related groupings reflecting medical interests were identified and are used to address practices and costs across institutions. Randomized control trials are conducted to evaluate treatment protocols, medications, and other aspects of medical practice.

Nursing has not been as successful as medicine in following this route. The most obvious reason being that the models used by medicine to accomplish evidence-based practice have limited usefulness for nursing. Medicine is concerned with the diagnosis and treatment of disease/pathological states. Nursing is concerned with management of health-related conditions. Understanding the components of the diagnostic process and the changing status of their interrelationships is more informative for nursing purposes than a diagnostic statement. The access to the information of concern to the discipline of nursing has not and is not as readily available to nursing as it is to some of the other health-related disciplines.

Nursing is often described as an invisible entity, its contribution to society recognized but difficult to describe. Countless workload measurement scales have been developed but they have had limited utility as they have not grasped the fullness of the entity known as nursing. Quality of nursing services has been measured by what can be called surrogate measures—decrease in falls, incidence of pressure sores. Now, electronic medical health records are being developed. If properly developed, can these be helpful in making nursing more visible and assisting nurses to articulate discipline specific information and best practices?

Initial efforts at building an electronic patient data base began with data associated with diagnostic related groupings, costing of associated services, admission-discharge data, controlling costs using length of stay information, developing budgets, developing work-load measurement indexes. Physician order-entry-recording- reporting systems including reporting of diagnostic tests have been developed. Pharmaceutical delivery systems, administration and recording of patient medications, prescription services, detailed information about drugs including recommended uses and dosages, side-effects and interactions have been made available at point of service. For the most part these have been quite useful to health care administrators. Twenty years later, diagnostic related groupings are still used in determining payment scales for in-patient hospital services although repeated studies have shown that these do not reflect nursing intensity. Nursing intensity has been shown to be a significant influence on actual costs and have been identified as a valid predictor of hospital charges, length of stay, and mortality (Welton & Halloran, 2005).

The first information systems developed within the health care industry supported the coordinating function of nursing—the most visible component of nursing practice. These included physician order-entry-recording systems, laboratory reporting systems, medication administration systems, patient admission-discharge systems, and to a limited extent from a nursing perspective costing systems. They might be helpful in reducing over-all service delivery costs and reducing system errors but is that all that quality of nursing is about?

The next generation of information systems has the potential to enable service providers to examine quality of nursing care in respect to specific procedures carried out, gross changes in patient status, number of falls, number of persons developing decubitus ulcers, and as so on (Liu, Castle, & Diesel, 2010). Again, the question must be asked—are these legitimate indicators of the quality of nursing and best nursing practices?

From work related to self-care deficit nursing theory, we know that the practice of nursing involves a constant comparison of relationships among conditioning factors, self-care agency, self-care demand, and the requirements for nursing. The information system associated with the development of electronic health records should be able to support evidence-based practice by providing a means for entering, analyzing, and extracting data relative to these elements and which supports the processes associated with day-to-day decision making of nurses as they interface with persons requiring their services.

In an effort to capture the essence of nursing, one set of researchers developed what they termed a domain model of the nursing process (Goosen et al., 2004). They indicate that to be useful, such modeling requires input from clinicians regarding workflow and content. There have been numerous data sets developed which purport to reflect the concerns of nursing. For the most part these have been constructed from data reflecting what nurses are perceived to do—the tasks they are performing and the problems they appear to be dealing with. The cognitive processes in which they are engaging and the content related to those processes, the purposes to be achieved, and how they envision achieving those processes is not captured. The cry is repeated in the literature—these data sets are more satisfying to the persons developing them than to the nurses caring for the patients.

Another group of researchers write "as nurses construct their records they make visible selected nursing elements, while other aspects of nursing become, or remain, invisible simply by virtue of what is and is not documented" (Kennedy & Hannah, 2007, p. 71). They also found in the review of a purposive sampling of records representing acute care, mental health, home care, and long-term care using ICN Nursing Practice Standards as a reference, the documentation was a task orientation and biomedical perspective. This is not to say that nurses have not been involved in development of these data sets or that nurses have not been involved in efforts to merge data sets—for example, those related to nursing diagnosis classifications and nursing intervention classifications. They have. But these lists have been developed without first specifying the proper object of nursing, then identifying the elements of concern within that proper object and developing some understanding of how the elements are related to one another and the meaning they have for nursing practice—how the elements are understood and expressed in nursing practice situations. Without this understanding there is only limited basis for specifying the components which should be included in an electronic nursing record and capturing the essence and components of nursing practice which are not apparent from analysis of current medical/nursing records or observation of nursing activities. Completeness of this record is fundamental to exploring and establishing desirable outcomes of nursing practice, for evaluating degree of achievement of those outcomes, and for establishing an evidence-based nursing practice.

Between the work of the Nursing Development Conference Group (NDCG) and the establishment of the Orem Study Group in 1993, a small group of nurses began meeting two or three times a year with Dorothea Orem to explore the utility of self-care deficit nursing theory as a framework for developing an electronic nursing information system (Bliss-Holtz, Taylor, & McLaughlin, 1992). This work resulted in detailing of the content associated with the processes of nursing—diagnosis and planning, design and production, control and evaluation. Included was a study which validated the processes and content associated with those processes in a sample of practicing nurses (Bliss-Holtz, Taylor, & McLaughlin, 1990). And then came the war known as "Desert Storm," which interfered with continued funding of this project to the implementation phase. However, the basis of this work, the link between nursing theory and development of a nursing information system, is still valid.

Nursing information systems have been developed by a variety of vendors. These have not proven to be universally useful and/or complete. The vendors are reluctant to have these information systems reflect a nursing theory base as they see these as having limited sales potential. Thus, the interests of the vendors are being served but not the interests of nursing. Although capturing data related to physiological indicators of health state, physician prescribed treatments, and some nursing treatments and patient responses may be generically useful, these systems fail to capture the complexity and totality of the concerns of nursing. A theory of nursing practice such as self-care deficit nursing theory and the related developments of the practice sciences can be useful in helping to develop a system which is more representative of the total essence of nursing. How can this theory be useful?

The focus of concern of nursing and the language to describe that focus of concern, to name the elements, has been specified. The nursing system has been identified as the product of nursing and the characteristics of this system described. It has been identified that this system has social, interpersonal, and technological dimensions. It is comprised of the patient variables of self-care practices, self-care agency, and self-care demand and the nursing variable of nursing agency. Factors that condition these variables have been specified. The substantive structure of the data elements has been specified. The processes of nursing practice and the content of those processes has been theoretically and practically derived and described. The structure of the interrelationships of the content elements is available for use in designing the structure for information processing.

The development of an electronic record is a two edge sword. Though it can contribute to the development of nursing science and nursing knowledge, it can also inhibit that development. The data elements identified for inclusion and the processes for manipulation of that data exert a powerful influence on the focus of the nurse. Will it be concentrated on the processes of self-care, the abilities required to perform that care, and the interaction of those variables with conditioning factors or will it be on the conditioning factors—physiological signs and symptoms, incidence of falls, incidence of medication errors, and so on.

POPULATION-BASED PROGRAM PLANNING AND BEST PRACTICE GUIDELINES

Population-based program planning has been an integral component of public health services for some time with the nature of the population in large part representing particular medical diagnoses. Conceptualizing nursing services as programs for specific populations can also be useful to health care agencies which offer integrated services across several agencies and also in developing best practice guidelines. Designing such a service begins with establishing the focus of concern of nursing within the interdisciplinary health care organization. Direction for this comes from specifying the proper object, identifying the variables of concern to nursing and the interrelationships of those variables. The detail related to this process is the subject of Chapters 2–5. With this background work completed, the characteristics of the clinical population which are of interest to nursing and the focus of the service to be offered can be specified. Elements and relationships to consider include conditioning factors which are active in the specific sub-population, types of self-care limitations, interferences with requisites, component of therapeutic self-care demand. The following is offered as a beginning example of the impact of following framing the design of a program from a nursing perspective.

DESCRIBING THE POPULATION AND DESIGNING A PROGRAM

Describing the population begins with deciding on a main organizer that is appropriate. In the following example, the service being considered relates to persons who have to make lifestyle changes related to activity, diet, and following a therapeutic regimen to prevent exacerbations of chronic illnesses such as diabetes and heart failure. The following design is not complete but illustrates a process for developing a design framed from a nursing perspective incorporating what is known about the self-care system.

Population: Adults with chronic illnesses who are required to make changes in their self-care system in relation to diet, activity, and following a therapeutic regimen. These persons will require on-going access to a variety of services. They may require periodic hospitalization for diagnostic purposes or adjustments to the prescribed therapeutic regimen. For the most part these persons have low literacy skills, a range of cognitive impairments, and may or may not have a support person who can monitor effectiveness of self-care system.

Assessment of each individual should include the following.

1. Calculate components of therapeutic self-care demand and assess of self-care agency with emphasis on the following requisites:
   a. Maintaining a sufficient intake of food
      i. Dietary prescription should be clear, developed in accord with literacy and cognitive capability of the client/family
      ii. Determine extent of understanding of dietary prescription
      iii. Assess re ability to procure and prepare food
      iv. Evaluate adequacy of financial resources
      v. Assess impact of following dietary prescription on family system
      vi. Evaluate motivation to follow dietary plan
      vii. In cooperation with client, develop plan to monitor achievement of dietary goals
      viii. Evaluate client's understanding of indicators that professional assistance for diet planning is required

For diabetic patients a major component of the therapeutic self-care demand would be requisites related to preventing and monitoring self for complications. For example, the design should include specific cognitively and physically appropriate guides for foot care and monitoring of feet with instructions about when to seek help.

Also included should be specific directions for nurses to follow protocols related to monitoring feet, foot care, and treatment protocols.

Liason and follow-up for each individual.

1. Identify agencies which may be of assistance to the client and establish a referral/reporting system.
2. Provide specific instructions for client re when to follow up and with whom.
3. Establish tracking system re follow-up.

Table 9.1 illustrates a model for delivering nursing care across a continuum of community agencies.

TABLE 9.1
Nursing Care Management Across Continuum of Community Agencies

NURSING CRITERIA FOR DECISION MAKING	SUPPORTIVE-DEVELOPMENTAL NURSING SYSTEM IN-RESIDENCE CARE	SUPPORTIVE-DEVELOPMENTAL OR PARTLY COMPENSATORY NURSING SYSTEM AMBULATORY CARE	SUPPORTIVE-DEVELOPMENTAL, PARTLY/WHOLLY COMPENSATORY CARE INSTITUTIONAL OR IN-RESIDENCE CARE
Calculate therapeutic self-care demand	Home Self/dependent care	MD office, clinic, Surgicenter, and so on	Inpatient facility Home
Estimate adequacy of self-dependent care	Home—personal care Retirement community	Home health Day care	
Estimate values of basic conditioning factors that are operational Stability/instability Acuity/chronicity of health state Complexity of diagnosis and treatment Assess physical, social, cultural environment	Nursing home Hospice		
Estimate extent and urgency of other health services needed			
Specify type/amount of nursing needed; Estimate costs			

OUTCOMES

Before embarking on any program to determine effectiveness of a service, the outcomes to be achieved must be established and categories for data collection and analysis identified. Allison and McLaughlin-Renpenning (1999) reported on outcome categories reflecting data collected about variables of concern to nursing (self-management systems, self-care demand, self-care agency) that could be used to track data in the patient record which could be used to determine outcomes and to construct a data base to inform evidence-based decision making and evidence-informed practice. The categories are presented in Exhibit 9.1.

EXHIBIT 9.1
Self-Care Deficit Nursing Theory Outcome Categories

PATIENT
1. Self-management system
   1.1 Adequate or taking action to modify
   1.2 Integrated into a broader system of living
2. Therapeutic self-care demand (actions to meet requisites)
   2.1 Calculates:
      2.1.1 what needs to be done
      2.1.2 how—best methods to use
      2.1.3 time sequence
      2.1.4 equipment
   2.2 Adjusts as necessary
   2.3 Actions performed
      2.3.1 quantitatively—complete
      2.3.2 qualitatively—how well, consistency
3. Self-care agency
   3.1 General self-care agency
      3.1.1 developed
      3.1.2 exercised
      3.1.3 adequate
   3.2 Self-care operations performed
      3.2.1 knowing
      3.2.2 decision making
      3.2.3 acting
   3.3 Power components
4. Dependent-care system
   4.1 Adequate or taking action to modify
   4.2 Dependent-care operations performed
      4.2.1 knowing
      4.2.2 decision making
      4.2.3 acting

(Continued)

4.3 Development of dependent-care agency

4.4 Dependent-care system integrated into self-care system of dependent

4.5 Dependent-care system and self-care system of dependent integrated into daily living

4.6 Dependent-care system and self-care system of caregiver integrated into daily living

4.7 Cooperation and coordination between caregivers if more than one

5. Basic conditioning factors

5.1 Environment—conditions of living–managing/modifying

5.2 Health state/system factors—managing

5.3 Family system factors—managing/modifying

5.4 Personal sociocultural factors—managing/modifying

NURSING

6. Nursing system

6.1 Identified self-care limitations

6.2 Self-care deficits overcome, compensated for

6.3 Self-care agency maintained, protected

6.4 Self-care agency increased

6.5 Dependent-care system established, operable, adequate

7. Regulating/monitoring basic conditioning factors

7.1 Condition, prevention of complications

7.2 Therapy, effects, results

7.3 Bodily functions, elimination, etc.

7.4 Safe, protective use of equipment

7.5 Safe, protective, supportive physical, social, psychological environment

7.6 Coordination of communication with other health care services

7.7 Availability, adequacy of follow-up services

Source: Adapted from S. E. Allison and K. McLaughlin-Renpenning, *Nursing Administration in the 21st Century* (Thousand Oaks, CA: Sage Publications, 1999).

SUMMARY

In this chapter, the utility of a self-care deficit nursing theory to provide guidance for developing evidence-based decision making in nursing and evidence-based practice has been illustrated. Evidence-based practice begins with defining the domain and boundaries of nursing, specifying the variables of concern and collecting data related to those variables in a format that the data can be manipulated and analyzed. It also requires an organizational climate that encourages reflective practitioners and provides opportunities for nurses to practice reflectively.

REFERENCES

Allison, S. E., & McLaughlin-Renpenning, K. (1999). *Nursing administration in the 21st century.* Thousand Oaks, CA: Sage Publications.

Bliss-Holtz, J., Taylor, S. G., & McLaughlin, K. (1990). Validating nursing theory for use within a computerized nursing information system. *Advances in Nursing Science, 13,* 46–52.

Bliss-Holtz, J., Taylor, S. G., & McLaughlin, K. (1992). Nursing theory as a base for a computerized nursing information system. *Nursing Science Quarterly, 5,* 124–128.

Carper, B. A. (1978). Fundamental patterns of knowing. *Advances in Nursing Science, 1,* 13–23.

Geden, E., Isaramalai, S., & Taylor, S. G. (2001). Self-care deficit nursing theory and the nurse practioner's practice in primary care settings. *Nursing Science Quarterly, 14,* 29–33.

Goosen, W. T. F., Ozbolt, J. G., Coenen, A., Park, H., Mead, C., Ehnfors, M., et al. (2004). Development of a professional domain model for the nursing process for use within the health level 7 reference information model. *Journal of American Medical Informatics Association, 11,* 86–194.

Kennedy, M. A. & Hannah, K. (2007). Representing nursing practice: Evaluating the effectiveness of a nursing classification system. *Canadian Journal of Nursing Research, 39,* 58–79.

Liu, D., Castle, G., & Diesel, J. (2010). Does use of advanced information technology in commercial minimum data set systems improve quality of nursing home care? *American Journal of Medical Quality, 25,* 116–127.

Lomas, J., Culyer, T., McCutcheon, C., McAuley, L., & Law, S. (2005). *Final report—conceptualizing and combining evidence for health system guidance.* Ottawa, ON: Canadian Health Services Research Foundation.

Porter-O'Grady, T. (2010). A new age for practice: Creating the framework for evidence. In K. Malloch & T. O'Grady (Eds.), *Introduction to evidence-based practice in nursing and health care* (p. 16). Sudbury, MA: Jones and Bartlett.

Spenceley, S. M., O'Leary, K. A., Chizawsky, L. L. K., Ross, A. J., & Estabrooks, C. A. (2008). Sources of information used by nurses to inform practice: An integrative review. *International Journal of Nursing Studies, 45,* 954–970.

Upshur, R. E. (2002). If not evidence, then what? Or does medicine really need a base? *Journal of Evaluation in Clinical Practice, 8,* 113–119.

Welton, J. M., & Halloran, E. J. (2005). Nursing diagnoses, diagnostic related groupings, and hospital outcomes. *Journal of Nursing Administration, 35,* 541–549.

10

Education and Evidence-Based Practice

THE NATURE OF EDUCATION PROGRAMS

*T*here are, or should be, direct correlations between levels of education and levels of nursing practice. In the United States, nursing education takes place within the system of higher education. At the time work on nursing theory was beginning, the predominant locus for nursing education was the hospital. Baccalaureate nursing programs were being developed in senior colleges and universities. Practical/vocational nursing education was becoming more common. The federal government identified a need for standardization in the education and practice parameters for practical nurses. As part of a project in the Department of Health, Education, and Welfare (DHEW), Orem developed *Guidelines for Developing Curricula for the Education of Practical Nurses* (1959). It presented the first nursing theory-based curriculum, albeit a rudimentary theory. This was the nucleus of Orem's self-care deficit nursing theory. What was unique was that the conceptual framework for the knowledge component was constructed before the curriculum was proposed.

Within a decade technical nursing education at the level of the Associate Degree was developing and there was a movement away from hospital-based diploma nursing programs bringing more nursing education programs within the system of higher education. More baccalaureate nursing programs were opening in liberal arts colleges, free-standing degree programs, and senior universities. Graduate programs were expanding at both masters and doctoral levels. Many educators, within and outside nursing, desired a seamless nursing education system with articulation from one level of education to another, from the licensed vocational/practical nurse to the nurse with doctoral preparation. This is still a goal for some.

Each of these changes in the educational system came with its set of controversies, some philosophical and many political within the profession and the academy and with the relationship of the profession to the health care system. There were questions of power and control of the practice of nursing. And there were questions as to the nature of the discipline and its place in academia. What level of education is appropriate at entry-level for professional nursing, for licensure? What are the differences in program outcomes? What are the appropriate graduate degrees: MS, MSN, MN, NP and PhD, DN, DNS, DNP? Can a seamless program, from LPN to the doctoral degree, be constructed such that the transition from vocational-technical education to professional education creates a change in the student's view of self as a nurse? What are differences between preservice education (preparation for licensure or work or entry into practice) and post-graduate nursing education in content and outcomes? How does this relate to changes occurring in society, health care delivery, and the content of scientific knowledge? And what does evidence-based practice mean for nursing education?

Logically levels of education and expected outcomes should be correlated with levels of practice and the work of nurses. Types of registration, licensing, and credentialing should also be differentiated. At this time in the United States as in some Canadian provinces, there are three legal distinctions. First is the vocational-technical level of LPN designed to prepare persons for limited nursing practice; though in reality these limits are not always discernible. All other graduates-associate degree, baccalaureate, masters—become registered nurses with an unlimited license to practice nursing but with limitations in associated medical practices. A few state jurisdictions have moved to requiring a bachelor's degree for entry to practice. Others have differentiated advanced nursing practice by requiring a different credential related to formal and continuing education; the major difference being less in the definition of professional nursing and more in the relationship of these practitioners to the field of medicine.

Significant changes have occurred in the education sector. There are now many more doctoral nursing programs than there were only 30 years ago. Clarification in the differences of the various doctoral education outcomes will, over time, lead to changes in masters education and baccalaureate education. All of these changes will depend on continuing clarification of the meaning and roles of professional nursing. The World Health Organization (WHO) proposed a set of global standards for nursing education in 2009 that have a goal that nursing education programs are based on evidence and competency. They note that three principles underpin all the standards:

1. Established competencies provide a sound basis on which to build curricula for initial education to meet health population needs.
2. The interaction between the nursing student and the client is the primary focus of quality education and care.
3. An inter-professional approach to education and practice is critical.

More specifically WHO recommends that graduates adhere to the code of ethics and standards of the profession. Some of the characteristics of the graduates of professional nursing programs are to use evidence in practice, possess cultural competence, to analyze and think critically, advocate for clients, and manage resources (Department of Human Resources for Health, 2009). The American Association of Colleges of Nursing (AACN) (2008) in the critical document Essentials of Baccalaureate Education for Professional Nursing Practice requires that "Professional nursing practice is grounded in the translation of current evidence into one's practice" (p. 3).

In 1966, Orem presented a clear and cogent analysis of professional nursing. It was her belief that, "Professionally educated nurses can move as a social force for the good of society but only when there is a corps of such nurses. The roles of the professionally educated nurse are:

1. To render nursing assistance to persons in situations where *creativity* and *flexibility* in the application of scientific principles must be utilized in selecting and applying ways to assist them in achieving health results through continuing therapeutic self-care. The creative use of nursing technologies is an essential part of this role. The nurse must be able to think scientifically and be able to bring theory to bear in observing the reality of nursing situations for which nursing technologies are unformalized, and in devising and applying ways to use nursing to aid in the accomplishment of health results.

2. To validate nursing technologies and to make them part of the body of knowledge that is nursing.

3. To extend the frontiers of nursing practice.

4. To develop the applied nursing sciences.

5. To transmit to others formalized knowledge basic to nursing practice through writing and teaching" (Orem, 1966, p. 21).

These roles clearly reflect the need for education that will enable the professional nurse to engage in evidence-based practice. Evidence-based practice will be a frame of reference for the professional nurse engaged in formal research or development of the nursing practice sciences. To have an evidence-based view of practice, the professional nurse needs to have a clear frame of reference regarding the proper object of nursing and the structure of the discipline to frame the problem.

Nursing is a practical science. In 1969, Simon proposed the science of the artificial. Artificial, meaning produced by art rather than nature, refers to things made by persons though not necessarily material, characterized in terms of functions, goals, and adaptations. Simon found the artificial to be "interesting principally when it concerns complex systems that live in complex environments" (p. xi). Simon's work provided NDCG with many other insights that aided them in their development of the theory of nursing systems and the science of design—which he called "the core of all professional training." Similarly, Argyris and colleagues were developing theories of practice and actions science (Argyris & Schon, 1974; Argyris, Putnam, & Smith, 1985). They presented ideas related to problem framing or setting; that is, when a problem is selected, we select what we will treat as the "things" of the situation and set the boundaries of our attention to it. We are able to impose upon the problem a coherence which allows us to say what is wrong and in what directions the situation needs to be changed (Schön, 1983, p. 40). Other important concepts introduced at that time were those of the interrelationship of scientist and practitioner, reflection, and learning. To some extent they were overshadowed by the increasing favor of the empirical sciences related to the natural, leading to a focus on the relevant nonnursing sciences as shown in Figure 1.4. The precepts of action science, the science of the unique and interpretive sciences are now gaining popularity as nursing and nursing education consider the nature of evidence, as described in Chapter 9.

As previously noted, the self-care deficit nursing theory provides a language for nursing. Every discipline has its own language elaborating the meaning of its phenomenon of concern, and the scholars of that discipline must know its unique language (Parse, 2001, p. 273). Students need to know from their first introduction into the field that the language of nursing is more than and different from the language of medicine and other disciplines. It is most important that students be provided with learning experiences within the curriculum that form their identity of *self as nurse*. "To build a nursing identity requires a deeper understanding and appreciation of the nursing theories and frameworks" (Senthuran, 2010, p. 245). This includes knowing and accepting the language of nursing and the types of evidence accepted within the discipline. It also necessarily includes the moral development of the student/person as nurse.

Baccalaureate students do not need to be analysts of nursing theories. They do need to know what it means to be a nurse from the perspective of the disciplinary structure and how to think critically within that structure. They do need to be critical thinkers. In the end, education for evidence-based practice must begin with critical thinking skills, a skill that the faculty must possess. They must be able to share and develop this with the students. There are many resources for critical thinking exercises. A simple one was developed by Johnson (2010) using five steps, with the acronym CRITO:

> state a Conclusion or claim, state Reasons or evidence meant to convince the reader, test the Inference, or argument, test the Truth of the reasons or evidence and construct the strongest imaginable Objections, and respond to them.

Another essential concept for developing the competence for evidence-based practice congruent with self-care deficit nursing theory is the concept of design. There are design and production operations described in Chapter 6. As a professional intellectual activity, design requires both practical experience and theoretical support. Mastery of a profession can only come through mentoring, coaching, and experiential learning as a member of a community of practice, in addition to the appropriate academic development of a leader throughout the course of a career. Banach (2009) described some critical elements of teaching the process of design to students, in both academic and practical settings, using leadership teams. Among the elements of the academic content, he identified as essential content the art of design, philosophy and design theory; systems-thinking lessons to establish an appreciation for relationships, creativity, complex adaptive systems, emergence, and self-organization. They focus on communications theory, organizational theory, and leadership along with the environment of design, integrating a study of edge theory, sense making, adaptive leadership, power and influence, and learning organizations to link the theoretical underpinnings to reflective practice. The academic course gives the students a deep intellectual foundation, preparing them to apply the design methodology to different and wide-ranging complex situations.

In practical exercises, students apply theoretical concepts, explore the art-of-design approach, lead operational planning teams, and develop their communication skills. Practical exercises cover the key elements of the design approach: receipt of situation, development of the environmental frame, problem frame, design concept, and design to planning. Students create an "environmental frame," "initial problem statement," and an "initial theory of action." They continue the learning begun in the first experience by generating "problem frame," "revised problem statement," and an "updated theory of action." The final practical experience gives the students the opportunity to design with the final outcome of the practical exercises being a translation of all learning achieved in the design methodology. It includes the creation of a "design concept" resulting in a formalized plan for action. These series of integrative experiences give substance to the academic subjects. An approach such as this might be more helpful to the professional nurse student preparatory to evidence-based practice than a focus on traditional research methods courses.

Before one can meaningfully talk about teaching methods for nurse education, consideration needs to be given to the structure of content and intended outcomes. The model of the structure of the discipline of nursing (Figure 1.4) gives guidance for the arrangement and selection of learning experiences and outcomes. Besides the structure of the discipline, the "content, processes, context, and environment" which are part of any complete nursing theory (Barnum, 1998) provide essential content for the curriculum.

The Essentials for Baccalaureate Nursing Education provides guidelines for what to include in a curriculum. It remains the prerogative of the faculty to determine the structure, sequence of courses, and learning experiences to meet these essentials. Although there is much written on pedagogy and using a variety of new technologies, instruction gains meaning from the curriculum. Nursing is a practical science. There are things nurses need to know and think about, they have a public or social responsibility to help people care for themselves. These are the substance of the curriculum and give guidance to teaching strategies.

Nursing is not a liberal art where the learner is concerned with critical analysis nor is it a natural science where the student learns the scientific method, mathematical models, and principles. It is all of these and more. The curriculum must be well designed to integrate all of these kinds of learning within the context of nursing practice.

The level of education must be used to give form to a curriculum and subsequently to nursing practice, and it is that level that affects engagement in nursing research and theory development and evidence-based practice. There are three basic levels of education within the profession. *Level 1* is concerned with the teaching of what to do, "certain limited skills and use of techniques necessary for task performance without much conceptualization as to where and how the techniques are derived." *Level 2* focuses on the "solving of practical problems in the profession so that a certain end product can be produced. It emphasizes information gathering to the extent that it is needed for the end product and emphasizes the use of techniques already validated." *Level 3* focuses on the "discovery of problems in the field and discovery of ways to solve them. It emphasizes creative thinking and demands development and validation of techniques" (Orem, 1968, pp. 51–52).

The Carnegie Foundation report (Benner, Sutphen, Leonard, & Day, 2010) on the profession of nursing focused on the developmental level of nursing education (2010). Taking an individual from naïve to potentially skilled practitioner of nursing, that is level 2 above, the proposed transformation focuses on the use of integrated nursing education-clinical practice modalities. The twenty-six recommendations made by the authors are all important. The recognition of the need to develop nursing skills within the clinical environment through new modes of learning is especially provocative. The challenge will be to keep the focus of the learning on nursing, nursing knowledge, and the sciences of nursing within an interdisciplinary work environment.

Curriculum is an important part of the process of identifying essential learning and then structuring that learning to ensure that the students gain the knowledge and competencies necessary for safe and ethical practice. The graduates are able to add to the sciences of nursing appropriate with their level of education. The essence of professionalism is both having a unique or special knowledge and the self-imposed obligation to serve the community. The Carnegie Report does an excellent presentation of the issue of ethics and moral development in practice. It gives little attention to the need for a unique or special knowledge. Nursing is described in terms of "the changing landscape of nurses' work" (p. 20) with need for "nurses working in highly technical arenas within complex health care delivery systems, managing and titrating all the major medical therapies delivered in the acute care hospital, as well as in ambulatory care facilities and the home" (p. 21).

WHERE DOES EVIDENCE-BASED PRACTICE FIT INTO THE ARRAY OF NURSING EDUCATION POSSIBILITIES?

All practice should be evidence based. The difficulty comes in the definition of evidence. It is becoming accepted that evidence in nursing is not limited to the empirical. See Chapter 9.

Baccalaureate education is the foundation for professional practice and for professional specialization in nursing through graduate study in the university (American Association of Colleges of Nursing, 2008, p. 22). LPN, and Associate degree programs should teach how to use evidence-based technologies and participate as members of teams to work to develop new technologies and gather data to help validate the techniques in use.

Newhouse, Dearholt, Poe, Pugh, and White (2008) uses a process referred to as the PET process (Practice Question, Evidence, and Translation) as an easy method to use and remember. They report that the guidelines have been used for undergraduate, graduate, and doctoral courses and meet the essentials of baccalaureate, master's, and doctoral education. The guidelines are developed for use at the baccalaureate level to enhance decision making, but also the model and tools have high utility at the graduate level (Instructor's guide, p. 2).

ISSUES IN EDUCATION FOR EVIDENCE-BASED PRACTICE

The student needs to be taught a spirit of inquiry, develop a healthy skepticism about information. They need to be given the tools for critical thinking in all things. In patient/client situations, the students need to develop these critical thinking skills into clinical decision making skills, assessing the person's therapeutic self-care demands, self-care agency, and selecting or designing nurse appropriate ways of interacting or intervening. Knowledge of the discipline of nursing is necessary if the graduate is to be truly interdisciplinary in practice. Without this disciplinary perspective, the graduate runs the risk of being subsumed into or remaining subservient to other professions, always a technician.

Brown-Benedict (2008) suggested that "perhaps due to an obstructed vision, we have not defined nor have we crafted a strategy to implement the educational and clinical experiences all advanced nurse clinicians must possess for comprehensive client care" (p. 454). Banks-Wallace, Despins, Adams-Leander, McBroom, and Tandy (2008) describe a course, Conceptual Structure of Nursing, that is concerned with conceptualization and theoretical analysis of nursing phenomena and critical analysis of nursing theories that assists students in exploring what counts as knowledge and how knowledge is developed in nursing, including historical and contemporary factors that influence the development of nursing as a discipline (p. 69).

The education of nurses in advance practice programs as proposed in the literature needs to be evidence based. Evidenced-based practice will thrive only when the practitioners are critical thinkers and leaders in the development of nursing sciences. It is not wise to develop separate courses on evidence-based practice other than for the techniques used to develop protocols. Similarly with research; the only way practitioners will be able to use research in the field is if they are taught to be avid consumers during their education. "Reading research is a habit that requires cultivation. If the habit is not established during professional socialization, it is unlikely to develop after graduation. Use of research is a clinical skill, not merely an intellectual indulgence" (Downs, 1998, p. 247).

Walker and Redman (1999) believe that while the "shift to theory-guided, evidence-based practice is necessary, one ingredient is missing: attention to reflective practice. To fully integrate evidence-based care into practice, we must make nursing practice reflective in nature."

As the students develop the sense of inquiry and knowledge of the discipline, they also need to understand the process of using evidence to guide practice. Initially the student will look at evidence-based protocols already in place at the institutions where they are getting their clinical experience. They can incorporate the national guidelines available through the clearinghouses or in literature in their care. Students in professional nursing programs do not need the same level of basic skill development that technical nurses do. Rather, they need the solid knowledge base and analytical abilities to assess the situation and creatively design nursing systems for individuals, families, and communities individually and as leaders and members of teams, intra and interdisciplinary.

The development of curricula formed within the self-care deficit nursing theory was described and evaluated by Taylor (1985) and Berbiglia (1991). Illinois Wesleyan School of Nursing has used the self-care deficit theory as the model for its curriculum; modifying it as experience and new knowledge require (Hartweg, 2000).

Like research, evidence-based thinking should be an integral part of professional practice. Nursing has developed beyond the point where separate courses on evidence-based practice and research methods will influence the practice. These approaches need to be integrated in each and every course and practical experience. Professional nursing education must continue to focus on thinking first and doing secondly.

SUMMARY

Evidence is an integral part of nursing education at all levels. The ground work for evidence-based or supported practice lies in developing critical thinkers and system designers. In practice, every time the cliché "we've always done it this way" is used, that practice or technique needs to be examined and validated using existing evidence or creating evidence. The structure of the discipline of nursing as described in this book provides a way to move the profession of nursing and the body of nursing knowledge forward in an integrated way.

REFERENCES

American Association of Colleges of Nursing. (2008). *The essentials of baccalaureate education for professional nursing practice.* Washington, DC: American Association of Colleges of Nursing.

Argyris, C., Putnam, R., & Smith, D. M. (1985). *Action science.* San Francisco: Jossey-Bass.

Argyris, C., & Schön, D. A. (1974). *Theory in practice: Increasing professional effectiveness.* San Francisco: Jossey-Bass.

Banach, S. J. (2009) Educating by design: Preparing leaders for a complex world. *Military Review, 89*(2), 96–104.

Banks-Wallace, J., Despins, L., Adams-Leander, S., McBroom, L., & Tandy, L. (2008). Re/affirming and re/conceptualizing disciplinary knowledge as the foundation for doctoral education. *Advances in Nursing Science, 31*(1), 67–78.

Barnum, B. S. (1998). *Nursing theory: Analysis, application, evaluation* (5th ed.). Philadelphia: Lippincott.

Benner, P., Sutphen, M., Leonard, V., & Day, L. (2010). *Educating nurses: A call for radical transformation.* San Francisco: Jossey-Bass.

Berbiglia, V. A. (1991). A case study: Perspectives on a self-care deficit nursing theory-based curriculum. *Journal of Advanced Nursing, 16,* 1158–1163.

Brown-Benedict, D. J. (2008). The doctor of nursing practice degree: Lessons from the history of the professional doctorate in other health disciplines. *Journal of Nursing Education, 47*(10), 454.

Department of Human Resources for Health, World Health Organization. (2009). *Global standards for the initial education of professional nurses and midwives.* Retrieved from WHO/HRH/HPN/08.6) http://www.who.int/hrh/nursing_midwifery/en/Global standards for the initial education of professional nurses and midwives

Downs, F. S. (1998). The rightful place of research in academia. *Nursing Outlook, 46*(5), 246–247.

Hartweg, D. (2000). Use of Orem's conceptualizations in a baccalaureate program: 1980–2000. *International Orem Society Newsletter, 8*(1).

Johnson, D. (2010). *Critical thinking.* Retrieved from href=http://www.au.af.mil/au/awc/awcgate/awc-thkg.htm#critical or http://www.mcla.edu/Undergraduate/majors/philosophy/crito/

Newhouse, R. P., Dearholt, S. L, Poe, S. S., Pugh, L., & White, K. M. (2007). *Johns Hopkins nursing evidence-based practice: Model and guidelines.* Indianapolis, IN: Sigma Theta Tau.

Orem, D. E. (1966). Nursing education, 1966–1967. In K. M. Renpenning & S. G. Taylor (Eds.) (2003). *Self-care theory in nursing: Selected papers of Dorothea Orem.* New York: Springer Publishing.

Orem, D. E. (1968). Levels of nursing education and practice. In K. M. Renpenning & S. G. Taylor (Eds.), *Self- care theory in nursing: Selected papers of Dorothea Orem.* New York: Springer Publishing.

Parse, R. R. (2001). Language and the sow-reap rhythm. *Nursing Science Quarterly, 14,* 273.

Schön, D. A. (1983). *The reflective practitioner.* New York: Basic Books.

Senthuran, R. A. (2010). Why ask why? *Nursing Science Quarterly, 23*(3), 245–247. doi:10.1177/0894318410371834

Simon, H. (1969). *The sciences of the artificial.* Cambridge, MA: MIT Press.

Taylor, S. G. (1985). Curriculum development for preservice programs using Orem's theory of nursing. In J. Riehl-Sisca (Ed.), *The art and science of self-care* (pp. 20–32). Norwalk, CT: Appleton-Century-Crofts.

Walker, P. H., & Redman, R. (1999). Theory-guided, evidence-based reflective practice. *Nursing Science Quarterly, 12,* 4.

Appendix A

A View of Nursing Theory Development

The history of nursing theory development has been chronicled by many authors (Alligood & Tomey, 1998; Meleis, 1997; Nicoll, 1992; Nursing Development Conference Group, 1973; Reed, 2008), and in the primary source works of the theorists themselves. Nightingale's writings are used to mark beginning of modern nursing (Meleis, 1997). Though this chronology is typically begun with Florence Nightingale, there were many nurses and others who developed the practice of nursing in earlier times and different places. Meleis (1997) identified Roffaida Bent Saad Al-Islamiah as providing for the East that which Nightingale did for Western nursing. She accompanied the prophet Mohammed in his Islamic wars. Like Nightingale, she organized women to care for the wounded. "They both focused on caring, healing, promoting healthy environments, and on training other nurses" (Meleis, p. 27). By being more inclusive in our readings, a less western-centric view of nursing's history and theory might emerge.

Nightingale wrote of the understanding of disease as a reparative process and that nursing ought to assist the reparative process. She also noted that the same laws of nursing pertain to the well and to the sick, and special knowledge is needed by nurses (Nightingale, 1859). These are some of the first nursing theoretical statements. From her observations of air, water, drainage, cleanliness, and light, she generalized statements about the health of houses and wrote a special section on that in her book. Nightingale's theoretical statements were relational but not explanatory. She could describe a situation well and predicted outcomes and reduced mortality rates. But she did not have the conceptual tools available to her at that time to address health phenomena by explaining how or why environmental factors such as noise from the chattering hopes of visitors and music, or the colors in varieties of flowers affected patient mood (Reed, 2008).

By 1917, the need for standardized education for nurses led the National League for Nursing Education (NLNE) to develop the standard curriculum (1917), a curriculum for nursing education (1927), and a curriculum guide for nursing education (1937). The nursing leaders at that time accepted Nightingale's proposition that nursing dealt with both illness and health, inside the hospital as well as at home. Nursing knowledge was logically derived from the medical and human sciences as they were known at the time (National League for Nursing Education [NLNE], 1917, 1927, 1937).

In the first half of the twentieth century, the knowledge content of nursing was the tasks which nurses were expected to perform (NLNE documents). The development of the body of nursing knowledge was hampered by the view of nursing as an art or as a set of tasks to be accomplished with knowledge derived from other fields, most notably medicine. The work of knowledge development is found mainly in textbooks.The first nursing journal, *The American Journal of Nursing*, began in 1900. Definitions of nursing were expressed and served for many years as the basis for nursing knowledge along with knowledge from other sciences and logical and intuitive application of those principles (Henderson, 1966; Orem, 1956). Socially, nursing and medicine were undergoing major changes that would intersect and diverge in ways unknown and that are still evolving in the twenty-first century.

The formal development of theoretical views of nursing began in the 1950s when nurses recognized a need to develop the science of nursing through research to meet the standards of a profession and gain a rightful place in academia and health care (Gunter, 1962). As nursing moved into the second half of the twentieth century, the approach to the development of the discipline changed. Nursing began to understand the need to develop and articulate the purpose and nature of its contribution to the health of persons. Furthermore, the higher education community had expectations of logically developed and justifiable curriculums for disciplines wishing to become members. This led to increased attempts to understand the knowledge structure and the substance that makes up the discipline of nursing. It became more important to the emerging profession that nursing education programs be able to justify their place in academia. This meant having a conceptual and theoretical knowledge structure that could serve as a base for the research and knowledge development that is expected within the academic setting.

At the same time, there were demands in the practice arena for using scientific principles to inform nursing practice. A process for making nursing judgments was adapted from the scientific method (Yura & Walsh, 1967, 1973). It became apparent to some that, though it is necessary to have a process, it is even more necessary that the end toward which that process is directed be known, that is, the object. Many nurses chose to use the conceptualization of basic human needs as the end or objective for the process (Yura & Walsh, 1978). Maslow's (1970) hierarchy of human needs became the content of nursing curriculum for many nursing educators (Young, Taylor, & Renpenning, 2001, p. 5).

As the quest for disciplinary knowledge and professional practice continued, the development of conceptual models and general theories of nursing was being undertaken. A conceptual model is "a network of concepts, in relationship, that accounts for broad nursing phenomena" (King & Fawcett, 1997, p. 93). A theory is the "narrative that accompanies a conceptual model, including description of the elements of the model and their relationships expressed in propositions. It is considered to be a general theory if it takes into account all instances of nursing" (Connections, pp. 4–5).

In 1950, there were many nursing scholars working on constructing models and theories of nursing. From the general nursing community there was immediate interest in a particular expression as the conceptualization if it met the needs and beliefs of graduate students, faculties, and scholars looking for ways to describe their work. Educational institutions, supported by the NLN, recognized the value of a conceptual framework for the structuring of curriculum and identifying the substantive content of instruction. Many schools adopted an existing model as a conceptual framework. Others chose to develop their own models. It was a time when the creative expression of faculty was valued. There became many competing models. The work of these scholars culminated in the publication of models or theories of nursing. Rogers (1961, 1970), Levine (1967, 1969), Roy (1970, 1976), Orem (1971), King (1971, 1981), Neuman (1982), and Johnson (1980) were the first to move beyond the defining of nursing to develop more formalized models or to explain the basis from which nursing science could develop.

The basic questions that they attempted to answer were, "what is the uniqueness of nursing, who is the nursing client, how do people behave or act on their own behalf and on behalf of others, and what is it that makes up the particular set of actions, processes or relationships that are nursing."

Each of the theorists mentioned above developed her conceptualizations of nursing as human endeavor or nursing science as human science (as opposed to physical or natural science). They differed in their approach to naming the object or focus of nursing. Orem conceptualized the object as the human person experiencing actual or potential limitations in their ability to care for themselves on an ongoing basis (Orem, 1970). Roy (1970) viewed the object of nursing to be the human as an adaptive system. Rogers (1989) proposed what has become known as the science of unitary human beings, that is, unitary, irreducible human beings and their respective environments. Levine (1967) expressed the object of nursing through four principles of conservation (1967); for Johnson (1980) it was the person as behavioral system. King (1971) identified human being as the basic element in dynamic interacting systems. Neuman (1982) developed a systems approach, viewing nursing from the perspective of system theory.

Nursing scholars began to analyze, critique, and evaluate these works. Since the publication of these works in the 1960s–1970s, the analysis, evaluation, and development of nursing theory took over the focus in scholarly discourse. Additional and alternative explanations of the structure and substance of the discipline were put forth. New approaches for substantive theoretical work were put forth by Watson (1979), Parse (1981), Newman (1982), and other theory developers.

Stevens (1979), Chinn and Jacobs (1983), Fawcett (1984), Meleis (1985), and others assumed the important role of theory evaluators. Each presented their perspectives on models, theory and theory development, and the methods of analysis and evaluation of theory. They developed and applied their criteria to the existing nursing theories or models such as Orem, Rogers, or Roy. There was debate as to the nature of theory and models in practice, of the meaning of discipline, and the value and appropriateness of certain models or types of models or theories, such as grand theory. (Dickoff & James, 1968, 1971; Donaldson & Crowley, 1978; Hardy, 1978, Walker, 1971). Nursing scholars and practitioners engaged themselves in knowledge development through theorizing and doing research to explain the substance and the structure of knowledge that form the discipline of nursing and informs the practice of nursing. The meaning of nursing theory and the relationship of theory or knowledge from other disciplines to nursing theory through the construction of middle range theory received much attention. One area of discussion focused on the meaning of nursing theory and its relationship to theory or knowledge from other disciplines. Another position suggested developing middle range theory using theory from other disciplines to explain nursing practice. Research is to be conducted to validate outcomes and produce evidence-based nursing. A third position is that the development of nursing science must be based in a discipline-specific model or theory of nursing (Orem, 1997; Fawcett, 1999).

In the twenty-first century, the analysis and development of nursing philosophy, theory, and science continues. The level of philosophical and scientific prowess is more sophisticated. For example, Doane and Varcoe (2005) fused theory and practice together in their concept of *compassionate action*. Chinn's (Chinn & Kramer, 2008) *praxis*, first discussed several years prior to this edition, denoted the transformative process of developing knowledge through critical practice. And Reed and Lawrence (2008) proposed a paradigm for practice-based knowledge development in the clinical setting. Theorizing in the twenty-first century reflects shifts in philosophy away from modernism toward postmodernism and post-postmodernism (or neomodernism) in which theories are no longer regarded as stable ideas that correspond to a higher truth, but more as conceptual systems of ideas that influence and are influenced by their context. "Although postmodernism decentered positivist and foundationalist notions of theory, theory nonetheless is still valorized as a prestigious activity across disciplines" (Chaiklin, 2004, p. 97). Neomodern views reflected in theory development include pluralism in sources of knowledge and methods of theory development; pragmatism balanced by assumptions about the mystery of life; belief in the capacity of human beings for innovation, agency, and well-being; an openness to change and critique; and, valuing local truths as well as broader philosophies for their perspectives on what is emancipating, good, and healthful, and other goals in nursing practice (Reed, 2006; Whall & Hicks, 2002). According to Reed, Rogerian thought (Rogers, 1970) is evident in the participatory and holistic perspectives underlying twenty-first century nursing theorizing. Parse has taken a leadership role in the development of her theory of human becoming. The journal, *Nursing Science Quarterly*, founded and edited by Parse is one resource for those who are interested in nursing theory and science. Newman's *unitary-transformative* worldview (Newman, Sime, & Corcoran-Perry, 1991) identified substantive focuses for theory development such as the person's inherent potential for self-organization, innovative patterning, and connection to the environment. Cowling (2007) operationalized Rogerian philosophy in his description of participatory action research, which united researchers, if not practitioners, and patients in the quest for nursing knowledge. Reed notes that action is a reality of practice. So, though practitioners may face added challenges in practice-based theory development, it may be found that their action orientation provides distinct advantages over traditional approaches to theorizing. This view is consonant with that of Orem, whose work has always reflected the essential dimensions of action and of practice.

In 2004 Beckstead and Beckstead examined twenty nursing theorists for their use of theories from other fields suggesting some convergence of these helps us to understand the origins and trajectories of nursing theory in the twentieth century. Nursing theory development is described as "the work of creative minds" (Beckstead & Beckstead, 2004, p. 113).

Though it is interesting to see some shared knowledge, it is presumptuous to think that the theories developed primarily from views of knowledge of other disciplines. There was much nursing knowledge known to scholars and practitioners. It lacked organization and shared language. The works of which of these twenty—or more—theorists will stand the test of time is to some extent dependent on the endeavors of scholars, researchers, and practitioners. The development of communities of scholars, researchers, and practitioners working within one explicit model or theory will do much to advance the discipline and profession of nursing.

REFERENCES

Alligood, M. R., & Tomey, A. M. (1998). *Nursing theory: Utilization and application.* St. Louis, MO: Mosby.

Chaiklin, H. (2004). Problem formulation, conceptualization, and theory development. In A. R. Roberts & K. R. Yeager (Eds.), *Evidence based practice manual: Research and outcome measures in health and human services* (pp. 95–101). New York: Oxford University Press.

Chinn, P., & Jacobs, M. (1983). *Theory and nursing: A systematic approach.* St. Louis, MO: Mosby.

Chinn, P. L., & Kramer, M. K. (2008). *Integrated theory and knowledge development in nursing* (7th ed.). St. Louis, MO: Mosby.

Cowling, W. R. (2007). A unitary participatory vision of nursing knowledge. *Advances in Nursing Science, 30,* 61–70.

Dickoff, J., & James, P. (1968). On theory development in nursing: A theory of theories. *Nursing Research, 17*(3), 197–203.

Dickoff, J., & James, P. (1971). Clarity to what end? *Nursing Research, 20*(6), 499–502.

Doane, G. H., & Varcoe, C. (2005). Toward compassionate action: Pragmatism and the inseparability of theory/practice. *Advances in Nursing Science, 28,* 81–89.

Donaldson, S. K., & Crowley, D. M. (1978). The discipline of nursing. *Nursing Outlook, 26*(2), 113–120.

Fawcett, J. (1984). *Analysis and evaluation of conceptual models of nursing.* Philadelphia: Lippincott.

Fawcett, J. (1999). The state of nursing science: Hallmarks of the 20th and 21st centuries. *Nursing Science Quarterly, 12,* 311–315.

Gunter, L. M. (1962). Notes on a theoretical framework for nursing research. *Nursing Research, 11*(4), 219–222.

Hardy, M. (1978). Perspectives on nursing theory. *Advances in Nursing Science, 1*(1), 37–48.

Henderson, V. (1966). *The nature of nursing.* New York: Macmillan Publishing.

Johnson, D. E. (1980). The behavioral systems model for nursing. In J. P. Reihl & C. Roy (Eds.), *Conceptual models for nursing practice* (2nd ed.). New York: Appleton-Century-Crofts.

King, I. M. (1971). *Toward a theory for nursing.* New York: John Wiley & Sons, Inc.

King, I. M. (1981). *A theory for nursing.* New York: John Wiley & Sons.

King, I. M., & Fawcett, J. (Eds.). (1997). *The language of nursing theory and metatheory.* Indianapolis, IN: Sigma Theta Tau International Center Nursing Press.

Levine, M. E. (1967). The four conservation principles of nursing. *Nursing Forum, 61*(1), 45.

Levine, M. E. (1969). *Introduction to clinical nursing.* Philadelphia: F. A. Davis.

Maslow, A. H. (1970). *Motivation and personality.* New York: Harper & Row.

Meleis, A. (1985). *Theoretical nursing: Development and progress.* Philadelphia: Lippincott.

Meleis, A. I. (1997). *Theoretical nursing: Development and progress.* (3rd ed.). Philadelphia: Lippincott.

National League of Nursing Education (1917, 1927, 1937). *A curriculum guide for schools of nursing.* New York: National League of Nursing Education.

Neuman, B. (1982). *The Neuman systems model: Application to nursing education and practice.* Norwalk, CT: Appleton-Century-Crofts.

Newman, M. (1982). *Health as expanding consciousness.* New York: National League for Nursing Press.

Newman, M. A., Sime, A. M., & Corcoran-Perry, S. A. (1991). The focus of the discipline of nursing. *Advances in Nursing Science, 14,* 1–6.

Nicoll, L. (1992). *Perspectives on nursing theory.* Philadelphia: Lippincott.

Nightingale, F. (1969). *Notes on nursing: What it is, and what it is not.* New York: Dover. (Original work published 1859).

Nursing Development Conference Group. (1973). *Concept formalization in nursing: Process and product.* Boston: Little Brown & Co.

Orem, D. E. (1956). The art of nursing in hospital nursing services: An analysis. In K. M. Renpenning & S. G. Taylor (Eds.), *Self-care theory in nursing: Selected papers of Dorothea Orem.* New York: Springer.

Orem, D. E. (1997). Views of human beings specific to nursing. *Nursing Science Quarterly, 10*(1), 26–31.

Orem, D. E. (1970). *Foundations of nursing.* Privately published.

Orem, D. E. (1971). *Nursing: Concepts of practice.* New York: McGraw-Hill.

Parse, R. R. (1981). *Man-living-health: A theory of nursing.* New York: John Wiley & Sons.

Reed, P. G. (2006). Neomodernism and evidence based nursing: Implications for the production of nursing knowledge. *Nursing Outlook, 54*(1), 36–38.

Reed, P. (2008). Practitioner as theorist: A reprise. *Nursing Science Quarterly, 21*(4), 315–321.

Reed, P. G., & Lawrence, L. A. (2008). A paradigm for the production of practice-based knowledge. *Journal of Nursing Management, 16,* 422–432.

Rogers, M. E. (1961). *Educational revolution in nursing.* New York: Macmillan.

Rogers, M. E. (1989). *An introduction to the theoretical basis of nursing.* Philadelphia: F. A. Davis.

Rogers, M. E. (1970). *An introduction to the theoretical basis of nursing.* Philadelphia: F. A. Davis.

Roy, C. (1970). Adaptation: A conceptual framework in nursing. *Nursing Outlook, 18*(3), 42–45.

Roy, C. (1976). *Introduction to nursing: An adaptation model.* Englewood Cliffs, NJ: Prentice-Hall.

Stevens, B. (1979). *Nursing theory: Analysis, application, evaluation.* Philadelphia: Lippincott.

Walker, L. O. (1971). Toward a clearer understanding of the concept of nursing theory. *Nursing Research, 20*(5), 428–435.

Watson, J. (1979). *Nursing: The philosophy and science of caring.* Boulder, CO: Colorado Associated University Press.

Whall, A. L., & Hicks, F. D. (2002). The unrecognized paradigm shift in nursing: Implications, problems, and possibilities. *Nursing Outlook, 50,* 72–76.

Young, A., Taylor, S. G., & Renpenning, K. (2001). *Connections: Nursing research, theory and practice.* St. Louis: Mosby.

Yura, H., & Walsh, M. B. (1967, 1973). *The nursing process: Assessing, planning, implementing, and evaluating* (1st and 2nd eds.) New York: Appleton-Century-Crofts.

Yura, H., & Walsh, M. (Eds.). (1978). *Human needs and the nursing process.* New York: Appleton-Century-Crofts.

Appendix B

A Detailed Self-Care Requisite

THE REQUISITE

Maintain an intake of water adequate to:

1. Keep concentrations of water constant in the blood plasma, tissue fluids, and intracellular fluids by balancing water intake with water loss through all channels of elimination.
2. Prevent, alleviate, or control disturbances of water concentration in body fluids—blood plasma, tissue fluids, and intracellular fluids—using technologies with known or presumed validity and reliability that have become parts of the common culture or are within the domain of medical practice. In the absence of such technologies, advanced practitioners in medicine and nursing must proceed by using the most advanced knowledge in search for ways to prevent, alleviate, or control disturbances. These regulatory results provide an understanding that water is essential for the life of cells, tissues, and organs, and for life processes. These regulatory results contribute to the continuance of human life and to the integrity of functioning of human beings.

PROCESSES FOR MEETING THE REQUISITE

The structural model for meeting the requisite is expressed in terms of four invariant processes named to reflect the outcomes sought:

1. Having the resource water, that is, ensuring the availability of safe water ready for intake.
2. Having knowledge and maintaining awareness of the quantitative and qualitative specifications of water intake.
3. Taking water into the body.
    a. Operations for alimentary intake.
        i. Operations for oral intake.
        ii. Operations for placement of water in stomach.
    b. Operations for parenteral administration of fluids.
4. Determining adequacy of intake of water.

Each of the four processes can be conditioned by one or more basic conditioning factors. The nature of a factor, for example, developmental state and its conditioning effects on a process, taking water into the body, gives rise to specification for method of intake by route. Each of the four processes may be conditioned by more than one factor, and the same factor may condition one or more processes.

CORE OPERATIONS OR UNITS OF ACTION
FOR THE INVARIANT PROCESSES

Core operations were identified for each of the four processes. These core operations are viewed as invariant; however, they must be personalized; they must be brought into conformity with the conditioning effects of internal or external factors for the individual for whom the therapeutic self-care demand is being calculated. The operations structure each process. The core operations for processes 1 and 4 (described above) are presented below; they are examples of subsidiary processes.

Core Operations (action units)

Process 1: Operations specific to having the resource water.

> *a.* Locating a water supply and means for procuring water.
>
> *b.* Checking for water potability and freedom from harmful elements; treating water when necessary to make it safe for consumption or increased potability.
>
> *c.* Procuring water and having it ready for consumption at specific times.
>
> *d.* Protecting water ready for consumption from extraneous materials.

The foregoing operations must be adjusted to the location of the person in relation to supply, regularity and frequency of water intake, and amount consumed. Under disaster conditions or in locations where there is no centralized source of safe water, procuring water is a major undertaking. Information about available water and preparation to ensure safety may be needed under these conditions and when traveling to ensure a safe supply of water. When water is administered parenterally, the operations are directed to water solutions that have been or are being prepared for administration.

Process 4: Operations for determining adequacy of intake of water.

> *a.* Estimating or measuring the quantity of water intake by all routes during a specified time period.
>
> *b.* Estimating or measuring the quantity and concentration of urine output during a specified time period.
>
> *c.* Comparing water intake with urine output during a specified time period, identifying quantitative differences, and specifying the concentration of urine.
>
> *d.* Estimating or measuring (when possible) loss of body fluids through sweating, regurgitation or vomiting, diarrhea, and blood loss during a specified time period.
>
> *e.* Incorporating results of "d" with results of "c" for a total comparison.
>
> *f.* Determining the presence or absence of signs of dehydration and its effects on human functioning.

g. Determining signs of water intoxication, for example, when kidneys are diseased.

h. Monitoring the effects of water deprivation or loss of body fluids on blood volume, fluid and electrolyte balance of blood plasma, tissue fluids, and intracellular fluids. (Denyes, Orem, & Bekel, 2001 pp. 51–52)

REFERENCES

Denyes, M. J., Orem, D. E., & Bekel, G. (2001). Self-care: A foundational science. *Nursing Science Quarterly, 14*(1).

Index